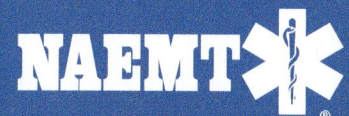

SECOND EDITION

All Hazards Disaster Response

Course Manual

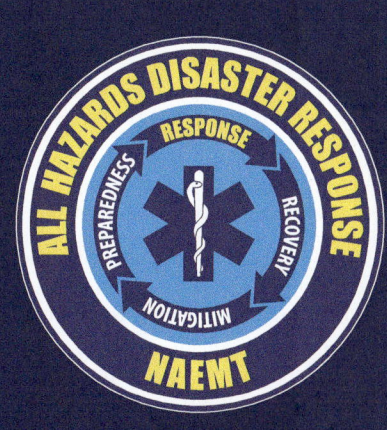

W0113349

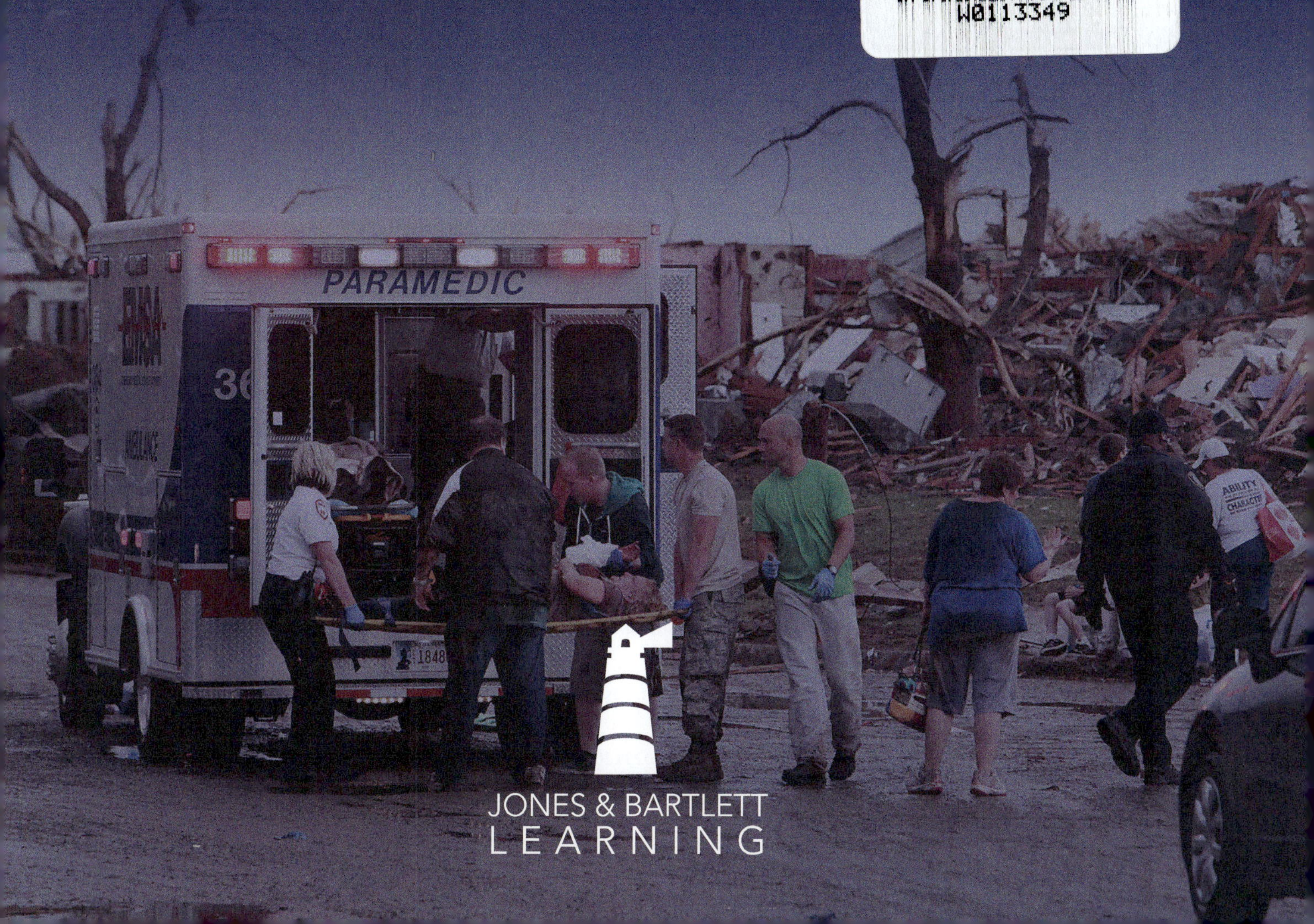

JONES & BARTLETT
LEARNING

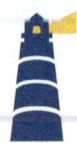

World Headquarters
Jones & Bartlett Learning
25 Mall Road
Burlington, MA 01803
978-443-5000
info@jblearning.com
www.jblearning.com
www.psglearning.com

Jones & Bartlett Learning books and products are available through most bookstores and online booksellers. To contact the Jones & Bartlett Learning Public Safety Group directly, call 800-832-0034, fax 978-443-8000, or visit our website, www.psglearning.com.

Substantial discounts on bulk quantities of Jones & Bartlett Learning publications are available to corporations, professional associations, and other qualified organizations. For details and specific discount information, contact the special sales department at Jones & Bartlett Learning via the above contact information or send an email to specialsales@jblearning.com.

29735-5

Production Credits

Vice President, Product Management: Marisa R. Urbano
Vice President, Content Strategy and Implementation: Christine Emerton
Director, Product Management: Cathy Esperti
Director, Content Management: Donna Gridley
Manager, Content Strategy: Tiffany Sliter
Content Strategist: Alex Belloli
Content Coordinator: Michaela MacQuarrie
Director, Project Management and Content Services: Karen Scott
Manager, Program Management: Kristen Rogers
Manager, Project Management: Jackie Reynen
Project Manager: Madelene Nieman
Senior Digital Project Specialist: Angela Dooley
Director, Marketing: Andrea DeFronzo
Senior Product Marketing Manager: Elaine Riordan

Vice President, International Sales, Public Safety Group: Matthew Maniscalco
Director, Sales, Public Safety Group: Brian Hendrickson
Content Services Manager: Colleen Lamy
Senior Director of Supply Chain: Ed Schneider
Procurement Manager: Wendy Kilborn
Composition: S4Carlisle Publishing Services
Cover & Text Design: Scott Moden
Senior Media Development Editor: Troy Liston
Rights & Permissions Manager: John Rusk
Rights Specialist: Liz Kincaid
Cover Image (Title Page): © David McDaniel/The Oklahoman/AP Photo
Printing and Binding: Gasch Printing

Library of Congress Cataloging-in-Publication Data
Names: National Association of Emergency Medical Technicians (U.S.), issuing body.
Title: All hazards disaster response course manual / National Association of Emergency Medical Technicians (NAEMT).
Description: Second edition. | Burlington, MA : Jones & Bartlett Learning, [2025] | Includes bibliographical references and index.
Identifiers: LCCN 2023049887 | ISBN 9781284297621 (paperback)
Subjects: LCSH: Emergency management--Handbooks, manuals, etc. | Disaster relief--Handbooks, manuals, etc. | Crisis management--Handbooks, manuals, etc.
Classification: LCC HV551.2 .A775 2025 | DDC 363.34/8--dc23/eng/20231205
LC record available at https://lccn.loc.gov/2023049887

6048
Printed in the United States of America
28 27 26 25   10 9 8 7 6 5 4 3

CONTENTS

CHAPTER 1 **Introduction** 1
Course Overview 1
What Is a Disaster? 1
Types of Disasters 2
   Mass-Casualty Incidents 2
   Natural Disasters...3
   Infectious Disease and Biologic Disasters.............................3
   Hazmat Disasters 3
   WMD Disasters 3
Comprehensive Emergency Management...4
   Prevention..4
   Mitigation..4
   Preparedness..4
   Response 5
   Recovery..5
References and Additional Resources..5

CHAPTER 2 **Incident Command System** 7
Overview of the Incident Command System......................................7
   Incident Command System 7
Characteristics of the ICS...8
Organization of the ICS 9
   Single vs. Unified Command..9
   Incident Command Post 10
   Command Staff..10
   ICS Sections and General Staff.......................................11
Disaster and Specialty Response Teams 12
   Types of Response Teams..12
   National Disaster Medical System and Disaster
    Medical Assistance Teams 14
Managing and Preserving Resources...15
References and Additional Resources...16

CHAPTER 3 **The Role of EMS in Disaster Response** 17
Goal of Emergency Medical Response to Disasters 17
Basic Steps in the Medical Response to Disasters............................17
   Initial Response...17
   Control Zones..19
   Triage and Treatment...20
   Transport..25
   Retriage 25
EMS Safety Principles in Disaster Response..................................25
   Situational Awareness..25
   Crew Resource Management...26
Psychological Response to Disasters...26
   Factors Impacting Psychological Response to Disasters.............26

   Signs of Psychological Trauma..................................27
   Psychological Response Interventions..........................27
  Physical Impact on EMS Practitioners..............................27
  References and Additional Resources..............................28

CHAPTER 4 **Mass-Casualty Incidents (MCIs)**.............................**29**
  General Considerations 29
   What Is an MCI?...29
   Key EMS Response Priorities During MCIs 29
   Fatality Management: Challenges for EMS......................30
   Patients with Special Needs...................................30
   EMS Challenges in Rural Settings.............................31
   EMS Challenges in Urban Settings.............................31
  Fires, Explosions, and Building Collapses...........................31
  Transportation MCIs..33
  Active Shooter/Hostile Event (ASHE) 34
   Personal Protection of EMS During an ASHE Incident 34
   Basics of Zones of Care 35
   Clinical Treatment Priorities: Direct Threat/Hot Zone 35
   Clinical Treatment Priorities: Indirect Threat/Warm Zone.........36
   Clinical Treatment Priorities: Cold Zone 38
  References and Additional Resources..............................39

CHAPTER 5 **Natural Disasters** **41**
  Types of Natural Disasters..41
   Warned Natural Disaster.......................................41
   No-Notice Natural Disasters 42
  Evacuation in a Natural Disaster 43
   Psychological and Social Impact of Evacuation.................43
   Phases of Evacuation 43
   Sheltering in Place vs. Evacuation 44
  Vulnerable Patients/Special Needs Population 45
   Identifying Vulnerable Patients..............................46
   Destination Determination 47
  Potential Hazards for EMS and Local Populations...................48
  Common Injuries 49
   Blunt Trauma...49
   Orthopedic Injuries 50
   Crush Injuries/Crush Syndrome................................50
   Exacerbation of Medical Conditions 50
  Triage and Transport in Natural Disasters 50
  Patient Tracking...51
  Public Education...51
  Preparedness 51
   Personal Preparedness 51
  References and Additional Resources..............................55

CHAPTER 6 **Infectious Diseases and Biologic Disasters** **57**
  General Considerations 57
   Disease Outbreak Terminology 57
   Models of Infectious Disease Transmission.....................58
   Controlling Infectious Disease Transmission...................59
   Personal Protective Equipment (PPE) 60
   Decontamination..64
   Ambulance Modification 64

Bioterrorism and Disasters 64
    What Makes a Biologic Agent a Bioterrorism Agent? 65
    CDC Risk Categories for Bioterrorism Agents 65
EMS Response: Infectious Diseases and Biologic Disasters 66
    EMS Practitioners and Bioterrorism 66
    General EMS Response: Concentrated Biohazard
       Agent vs. Infected Patient 66
    How Is Biologic Triage Different? 66
    Specific Steps to Prevent Infection 67
EMS Management of Specific Biohazard Agents 68
    Anthrax 68
    Plague 68
    Smallpox 69
    Ebola Virus 70
    Botulinum Toxin 71
Pandemic Preparedness and Response: Crisis Standards
    of Care 72
Case Study 73
References and Additional Resources 76

CHAPTER 7   **Chemical and Radiologic/Nuclear Disasters** **79**
What Are Hazardous Materials? 79
Similarities Between Management of Hazmat Disasters 79
    Hazmat Incident Identification 79
    Time of Dispatch 80
    Approaching the Hazmat Scene 80
    Chemical Placards 80
    Regulatory Agency Notification 82
    Zones of Operation 82
    Personal Protective Equipment (PPE) 83
    Decontamination 84
Chemical Disasters 85
    Classification of Chemical Agents and Toxidromes 85
    Type of Exposure 87
    Primary and Secondary Contamination 87
    EMS Considerations in the Management of Chemical
       Disasters 88
    Transport Considerations 92
Radiologic/Nuclear Disasters 92
    Types of Ionizing Radiation 92
    Disaster Scenarios 93
    Types of Radiologic Weapons 95
    Diagnosing Radiation Exposure 95
    Understanding Radiation Exposure 95
    Preventing Untoward Effects from Radiation Exposure 95
    Dose Rate Meters and Radiation Surveys 96
    Principles of Management and Decontamination 96
    Transport Considerations 96
Case Study 97
References and Additional Resources 100

CHAPTER 8   **Explosions and Blast Injuries** **103**
General Considerations 103
    The Many Causes of Explosions 103
    Closed- vs. Open-Space Explosions 103

The Imperative of Situational Awareness 104
Law Enforcement Interface 104
Triage Considerations 104
Transport Considerations 105
Special Populations 105
Explosives 105
Categories of Explosives 105
Explosion Terminology 106
Mechanisms of Injury 106
Types of Blast Injuries 106
Blast Lung Injury (BLI) 107
Tympanic Membrane Rupture 109
Abdominal Injuries
(Blast Abdomen) 109
Head Injuries 109
Multisystem Trauma 110
Crush Injuries 110
Compartment Syndrome 110
Incendiary Agents 111
Thermite 111
Magnesium 111
White Phosphorus 111
References and Additional Resources 112

GLOSSARY 113

INDEX 119

FOREWORD

Writing this foreword for the second edition of the NAEMT *All Hazards Disaster Response (AHDR)* course manual is an honor and privilege. Notably, the course addresses the challenges of responding to all threats, including no-notice and long-term manmade and natural disasters.

With the increased frequency and severity of disasters, including extreme weather-related ones, we can no longer leave disaster preparedness and response solely to disaster experts or the incident commander. Every EMS practitioner needs to be able to respond to any disaster at a moment's notice, just like they have always done. With the many challenges to our current disaster response readiness, each individual plays a critical role. Thus, our national preparedness is the shared responsibility of all levels of government, private and nonprofit sectors, and individuals.

The AHDR course focuses on EMS's role in supporting capabilities required for health care to save lives and maintain function during a disaster, including incident management and coordination, information management, patient movement and distribution, workforce, resources, operational continuity, specialty care, and community integration.

EMS practitioners have responded to previously unimaginable disasters, such as the September 11th attacks, the 2017 Route 91 Harvest Festival Las Vegas shooting, and the COVID-19 pandemic. Some disasters have had no prior response plans, training, exercises, or protocols specific to those disasters. EMS clinicians became real-time problem solvers for each of those elements and others. Given the threats we face, a critical skill set for each EMS practitioner is real-time problem-solving, adapting, and applying critical thinking rather than relying on protocols alone. Problem-solving requires a laser-like focus to identify and act on what it will take to save lives and protect the health care workforce during disaster response; if the solution doesn't work, adapt and find a better one.

Before the COVID-19 pandemic, many believed that the role of EMS in mitigating surges at hospitals was important. In a 2021 study, the National Institutes of Health (NIH) reported that nearly 1 in 4 COVID-19 deaths was potentially attributable to hospital strain conditions caused by surging caseload. Load balancing of patients among hospitals to distribute patient surges at those hospitals can literally be lifesaving. EMS practitioners, including those involved in interfacility transport, played a critical role in the load balancing of patients among health care facilities. Planning a successful surge response at the EMS, facility, and regional level is foundational to our shared goal of saving lives.

To save lives every day and during and after a disaster response, we will need to fill gaps in health equity and access to care that continue to be challenging after the COVID-19 pandemic. EMS plays a vital role, and this course can help.

The EMS workforce is the foundation for any emergency medical response, including disaster response. We need a resilient, adequately-resourced, protected, trained, and supported EMS workforce that is fully staffed for daily needs and is ready to deploy during a response to provide safe patient care. While that may seem a distant goal today, continued efforts to support the EMS workforce, including through educational courses like this, are critical. If the medical director for the first edition of AHDR, Dr. Craig Manifold were with us, he would agree.

Richard C. Hunt, MD, FACEP
Senior Medical Advisor, Office of Health Care Readiness
Office of Preparedness
Administration for Strategic Preparedness & Response
U.S. Department of Health & Human Services

PREFACE

Disasters and mass-casualty incidents of all types are increasing in frequency and intensity every year. The number of environmental disasters, transportation incidents, acts of intentional violence, and structural collapses continues to trend upward. Weather events, such as hurricanes, are stronger, and the impact of weather and climate disasters is rising.

Ensuring an effective EMS disaster response is time consuming, requires significant planning and the coordination of multiple agencies, and presents unique medical considerations. The second edition of *All Hazards Disaster Response* is intended to prepare EMS practitioners and other first responders for their unique and necessary role in disaster response. The case-based lesson presentations in the course provide students with the opportunity for interactive discussion. Disaster simulations throughout the course challenge students to apply their knowledge to various realistic situations.

New Features

- Revised table of contents
- Updates to all chapters
- New case-based lesson presentations
- New disaster simulations

The AHDR author team and NAEMT hope you find that the information contained in this second edition's lessons, disaster simulations, and course manual enhances your knowledge about the variety of disasters to which you are called on to respond by better preparing you to do the greatest good for the greatest number of people.

Matthew Levy, DO, MSc, FACEP, FAEMS, NRP
All Hazards Disaster Response Course Medical Editor
Deputy Director of Operational Medicine
Associate Emergency Medical Services Fellowship
  Director
Associate Professor of Emergency Medicine
Associate Professor of Surgery
Johns Hopkins University School of Medicine
Baltimore, Maryland

ACKNOWLEDGMENTS

Course Authors

Debra L. Bell, MS, EMT-T, CCEMTP, NJ-CEM
Vice President and Trustee
Southern New Jersey EMS Collaborative
Richland, New Jersey

Rebecca Carmody, AAS, EMT-P
Master Instructor, Nevada
Fire Training Instructor
Clark County Fire Department
Las Vegas, Nevada

Chris Hadis, MS, AEMT/IC
State Inspector
Agricultural Emergency Preparedness and Response
Commonwealth of Massachusetts

Brian Simonson, MBA, NRP, CHEC
SERAC Trauma Coordinator, Trauma Services
Novant Health New Hanover Regional Medical Center
Wilmington, North Carolina

Course Medical Director

Matthew Levy, DO, MSc, FACEP, FAEMS, NRP
All Hazards Disaster Response Course Medical Director
Deputy Director of Operational Medicine
Associate Emergency Medical Services Fellowship Director
Associate Professor of Emergency Medicine
Associate Professor of Surgery
Johns Hopkins University School of Medicine
Baltimore, Maryland

NAEMT Editorial Director

Nancy Hoffmann, MSW
Senior Director of Education, Publishing
National Association of Emergency Medical Technicians

AHDR Course Manual Development Editor

Pooja Mehrotra, MSc
Education Editor
National Association of Emergency Medical Technicians

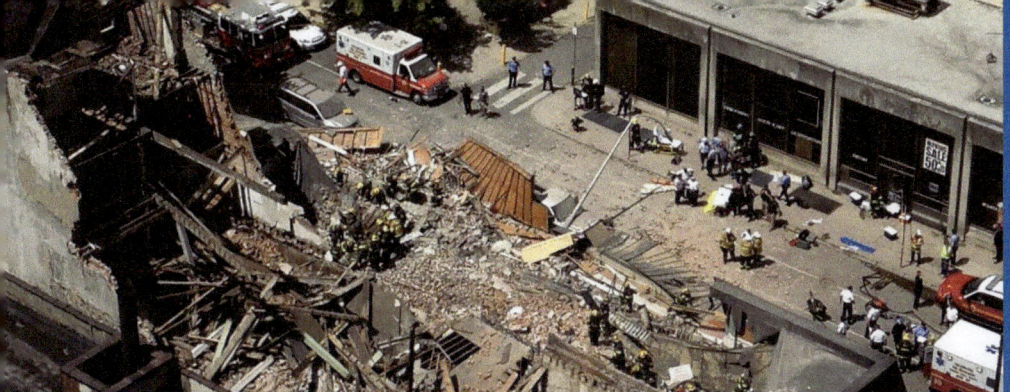

Introduction

LESSON OBJECTIVES

At the completion of this lesson, you should be able to do the following:

· Discuss the primary goal of the All Hazards Disaster Response (AHDR) course.

· Define the term *disaster* and list the types of disasters.

· State the guiding principle of disaster response.

· Describe the specific steps in comprehensive emergency management.

Course Overview

Welcome to the NAEMT's All Hazards Disaster Response (AHDR) course. This course has been developed by a team of disaster management faculty and subject-matter experts to strengthen practitioner preparedness and resilience when responding to all types of disasters. The course teaches students the principles and fundamental concepts of EMS response to disasters within an emergency response system. In addition, it highlights the considerations and best practices for assessing, triaging, and treating patients in all types of disasters, mass-casualty incidents, and public health emergencies.

The learning objectives for this course are as follows:

· Define the role of EMS within the incident command system.

· Explain how crew resource management and scene safety apply to EMS disaster response.

· Describe the role of EMS personnel during the different stages of a disaster.

· Discuss the components of EMS preparedness required to ensure that EMS agencies and practitioners are ready to respond to disasters.

· Describe the key processes associated with EMS operations during a disaster or public health emergency.

· Describe considerations and best practices for responding to patients in different types of disasters.

· Demonstrate the ability to incorporate best practices for EMS disaster response.

· Explain the critical actions required to support patient and practitioner safety during disaster response.

What Is a Disaster?

Disasters—whether natural or human-made, intentional or unintentional—are all too common (**Figure 1-1**). The United Nations reported 7,348 disasters worldwide from 2000 to 2019. These events killed 1.23 million people and affected more than 4 billion people, resulting in a global economic loss of US$2.97 trillion. The term *disaster* is used so frequently in everyday language that it is essential to arrive at a shared understanding of what constitutes a disaster.

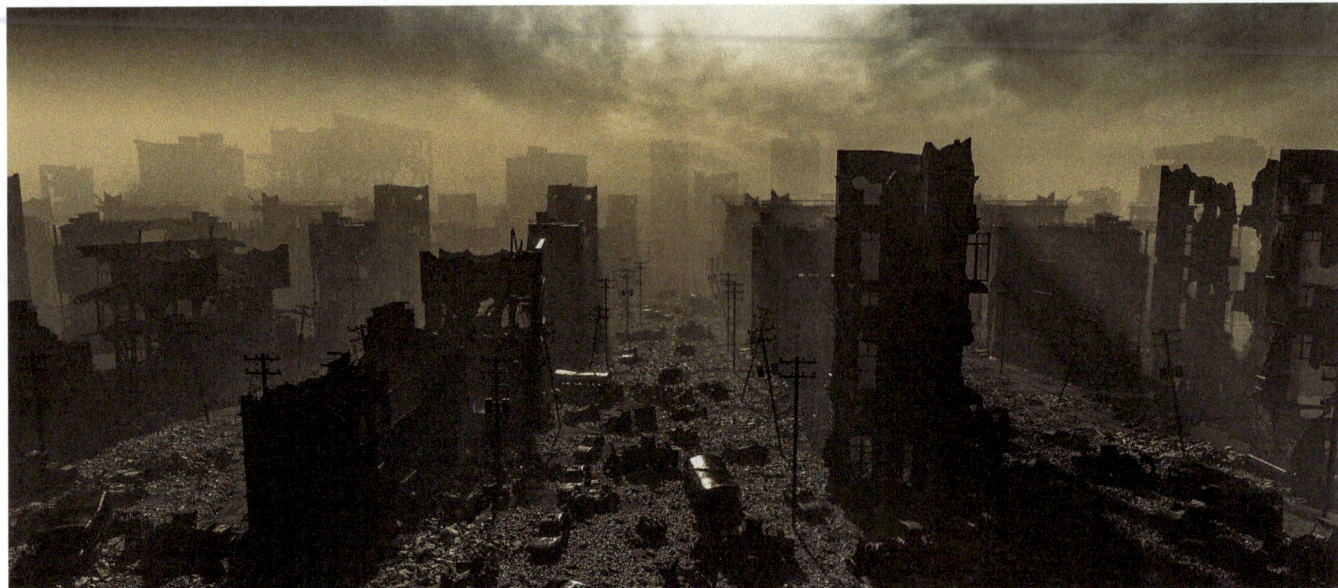

Figure 1-1 A disaster causes a serious disruption in services essential for a community, often leading to the prioritization of available resources to do the greatest good for the greatest number of people.
© santoelia/Shutterstock

The United Nations Office for Disaster Risk Reduction defines a disaster as "a serious disruption of the functioning of a community or a society at any scale due to hazardous events interacting with the conditions of exposure, vulnerability, and capacity, leading to one or more of the following: human, material, economic, or environmental losses and impacts." A disaster can also be thought about in terms of supply and demand. It is a situation in which the number of patients needing emergency medical assistance exceeds the capacity of the emergency medical system's resources, and thus requires additional, sometimes external, assistance. These definitions illustrate two key concepts:

1. The designation of *disaster* is not dependent on a specific number of victims.
2. A disaster exceeds the medical system's available resources and typically disrupts the system's infrastructure.

Disasters, by definition, disrupt the local medical and public health infrastructure. Although the degree of disruption, much like a disaster's timing, location, or complexity, cannot be predicted, a simple guiding principle of disaster medical response always holds true: Do the greatest good for the greatest number of people with available resources. This objective differs from "conventional" non-disaster-related medical care to do the greatest good for each patient. The concern for collective welfare extends throughout the disaster response and recovery phase, with the ultimate goal of returning the community to its level of predisaster functional status.

> *A serious disruption of the functioning of a community or a society at any scale due to hazardous events interacting with the conditions of exposure, vulnerability and capacity, leading to one or more of the following: human, material, economic, or environmental losses and impacts.*
> —United Nations Office for Disaster Risk Reduction

Types of Disasters

The framework of what constitutes a disaster supports many different types of disasters: mass-casualty incidents; natural disasters, such as hurricanes, wildfires, or flash floods; infectious disease pandemics; and incidents involving hazardous materials or weapons of mass destruction.

Mass-Casualty Incidents

In this course, the term *mass-casualty incident* (MCI) refers to a disaster that overwhelms the community's available resources. MCIs generate so many casualties that the available health care resources, or their management systems, are severely challenged or unable to meet the health care needs of the affected population. In other words, the number of patients exceeds the resources available, regardless of whether the incident is a motor vehicle collision, building collapse, airplane crash, natural disaster, infectious disease, biologic disaster, or hazardous materials disaster (**Figure 1-2**).

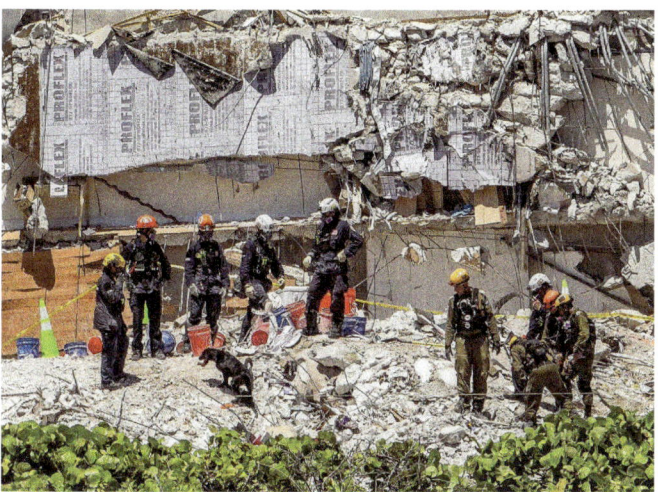

Figure 1-2 A mass-casualty incident overwhelms the community's resources.

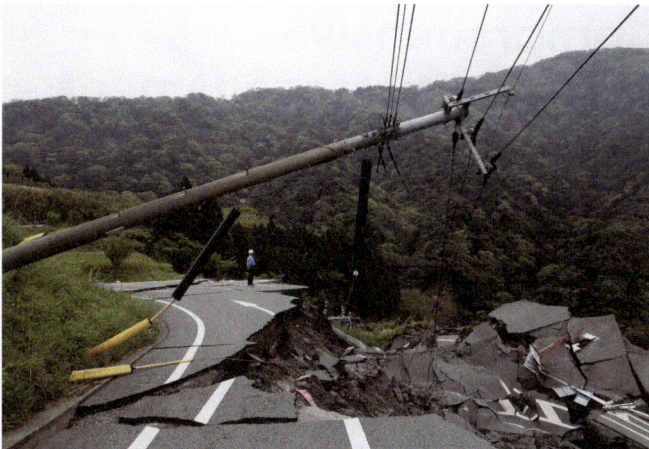

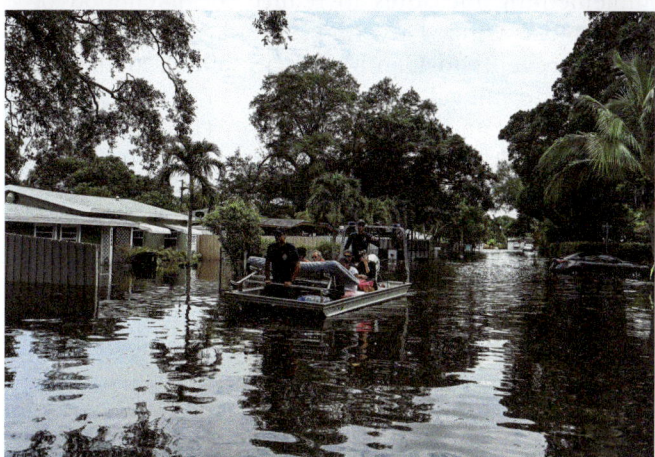

Natural Disasters

The U.S. Department of Homeland Security defines a natural disaster as any severe weather event with the potential to cause a significant threat to people, property, infrastructure, and homeland security. In addition to severe weather events, geologic events such as earthquakes, wildfires, floods, and volcanic eruptions are also examples of natural disasters (**Figure 1-3**).

Figure 1-3 A natural disaster includes any severe weather or geologic event that may cause a significant threat to people, property, infrastructure, and homeland security.

Infectious Disease and Biologic Disasters

Infectious diseases and biologic disasters involve biologic pathogens (diseases) that result in mass casualties. These include epidemics, pandemics, outbreaks of infectious disease, and bioterrorism attacks.

Hazmat Disasters

Hazardous materials (hazmat) can be found everywhere, including in vehicles, buildings, and homes. Hazmat disasters can be intentional or unintentional and may involve explosions or the release of flammable and combustible substances, poisons, or radioactive materials causing damage to property, infrastructure, and people (**Figure 1-4**).

WMD Disasters

A weapon of mass destruction (WMD) can inflict casualties of disastrous proportions. Although several different mnemonics are used to recall the various types of WMDs, the easiest to remember is **CBRNE**, which stands for **C**hemical, **B**iologic, **R**adiologic, **N**uclear, and **E**xplosive. History has demonstrated that WMD incidents, intentional or unintentional, can occur without warning anywhere.

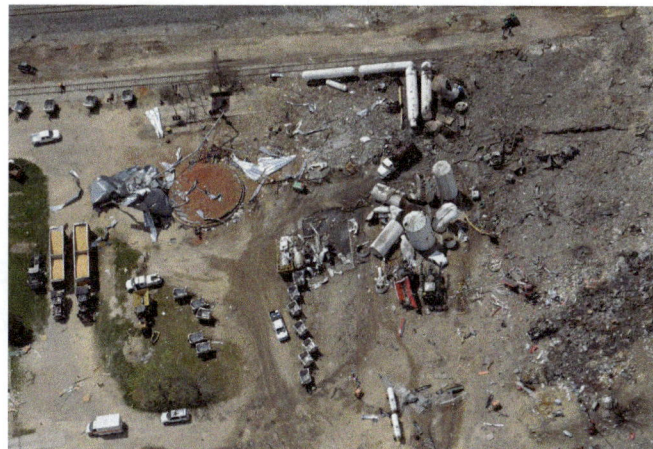

Figure 1-4 A disaster such as the derailment of a Norfolk Southern freight train in East Palestine, Ohio, in 2023 can result in the release of hazardous materials and disrupt communitywide infrastructure, such as power, transportation, and communications services.

Comprehensive Emergency Management

Comprehensive emergency management comprises the specific steps needed to prevent or manage an incident. This concept involves five components: prevention, mitigation, preparedness, response, and recovery (**Figure 1-5**).

Prevention

Although not all disasters can be prevented, **prevention** refers to proactively identifying potential hazards and implementing measures to reduce the likelihood of a disaster occurring. Prevention efforts must draw from previous events to identify system failures that can be corrected to mitigate future disasters. Prevention efforts may include safety measures, security checkpoints, public health education, and disease prevention.

Mitigation

Mitigation happens in the time between disasters, during which plans for response to potential events are developed and tested. It refers to actions taken to prevent or reduce the loss of life through structural and nonstructural measures. These defensive maneuvers may include such actions as fortifying physical structures, initiating evacuation plans, and mobilizing public health resources to mount a postevent response. Physical measures to mitigate a disaster could include moving trees away from a house, building flood levees, installing shutters, or installing metal detectors. Other disaster mitigation measures include amending or adopting new building codes, zoning requirements, buying insurance policies, or early warning systems for detecting severe weather.

Preparedness

Preparedness involves the advance identification of an incident and the specific supplies needed, including those to meet the needs of the population, such as durable medical equipment for persons with special needs; response equipment; personnel needed to manage the incident; and the specific incident action plan that would be employed if a particular scenario unfolds. Preparedness is a continuous process that includes planning, training, and educational activities for people, organizations, and communities if a disaster cannot be avoided. Developing preparedness plans (including special population considerations); conducting fire, tornado, and active shooter drills; identifying regional resources; and conducting joint training are all examples of preparedness actions.

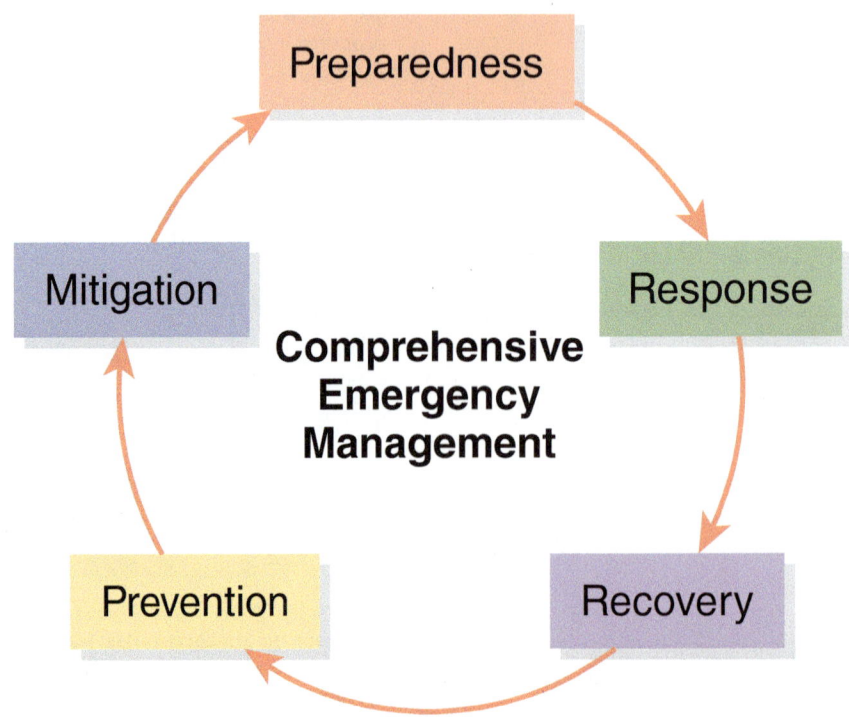

Figure 1-5 Steps in comprehensive emergency management.
© National Association of Emergency Medical Technicians (NAEMT)

Response

The **response** phase involves activating and deploying the resources to manage an active incident. Ideally, these resources were identified during the preparedness phase. Prehospital emergency medical practitioners typically operate during this period. The response occurs during and after the disaster and includes both short- and long-term actions. Measures are taken to minimize risks to life, property damage, and environmental loss. The appropriate response can help reduce otherwise preventable deaths. The skills of EMS practitioners, rescue teams, and medical support services are brought to bear to maximize the number of survivors of the disaster. Managing resources such as equipment, personnel, and supplies; implementing response plans; removing hazards; conducting search and rescue operations; and addressing the public are all examples of actions that take place during the response phase.

Recovery

The actions necessary to return the community to its preincident functional status (i.e., restoration efforts to return to normal or a new normal) happen during the recovery phase of the disaster. In the **recovery** phase, community resources are called upon to emerge from and rebuild through the coordinated efforts of the medical, public health, and community infrastructure (physical and political). The recovery process involves prioritizing essential services (food and water, utilities, transportation, and health care). It could include rebuilding damaged structures to new code specifications to reduce future risk or providing financial and mental health services for community residents. Recovery can take anywhere from a few days to several years, with some disaster recoveries spanning multiple generations.

SUMMARY

- A disaster is an event that causes a serious disruption in services essential for a community, resulting in crisis conditions. Often, medical services must prioritize available resources to do the greatest good for the greatest number of people.
- A disaster is not defined by a specific number of victims but rather by the disruption to community functioning due to hazardous events leading to losses and instability.
- Comprehensive emergency management defines the specific steps needed to manage an incident. It comprises five components: prevention, mitigation, preparedness, response, and recovery.

References and Additional Resources

Cuny FC. Introduction to disaster management: lesson 5–technologies of disaster management. *Prehosp Disaster Med.* 1993;6:372–374.

Public Health Emergency. 1.1: Mass casualty and mass effect incidents: implications for healthcare organizations. US Department of Health and Human Services. https://www .phe.gov/Preparedness/planning/mscc/healthcarecoalition /chapter1/Pages/implications.aspx. Accessed July 24, 2023.

Regan H. UN warns that world risks becoming "uninhabitable hell" for millions unless leaders take climate action. CNN. https:// www.cnn.com/2020/10/13/world/un-natural-disasters -climate-intl-hnk/index.html. Accessed July 11, 2023.

Starr GA, Allen TW, Stewart CE. Disaster medicine. In: Stone C, Humphries RL, eds. *CURRENT Diagnosis & Treatment Emergency Medicine.* 7th ed. McGraw Hill; 2011. https://accessemergency medicine.mhmedical.com/content.aspx?bookid=385&sectio nid=40357217. Accessed August 28, 2023.

United Nations Office for Disaster Risk Reduction. Disaster. January 18, 2022. Accessed August 28, 2023. https://www .undrr.org/terminology/disaster

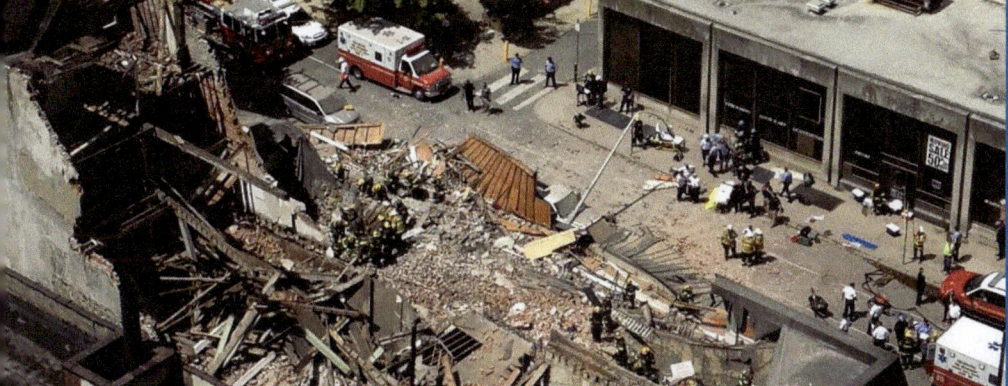

Incident Command System

LESSON OBJECTIVES

At the completion of this lesson, you should be able to do the following:

- List the characteristics of the incident command system (ICS).
- Describe the structure of the ICS and the function of each of its components.
- Discuss the different kinds of disaster response teams.

Overview of the Incident Command System

The **National Incident Management System (NIMS)** was developed to provide a template for a comprehensive nationwide, systematic approach to managing an incident, regardless of its cause, size, location, or complexity. NIMS offers a set of preparedness concepts for all hazards and events, outlines the essential principles for a standardized and consistent operating structure, and provides standardized resource management procedures. It utilizes the incident command system to oversee the direct response to a specific event.

Incident Command System

Many different organizations may participate in the response to a disaster. Therefore, effective management of a disaster requires an organizational structure that both provides a hierarchy of authority and responsibility and establishes formal channels of communication. The **incident command system (ICS)** provides this structure, allowing different types of agencies (e.g., fire, police, EMS) and multiple jurisdictions of similar agencies (e.g., city, county, state) to interface and work together effectively during a disaster response.

The ICS offers several important advantages during a disaster response:

- The ICS enables a standardized emergency response agency to operate more safely and effectively.
- A uniform approach facilitates and coordinates the use of resources from multiple agencies, working toward common objectives.
- Because the specific responsibilities and authority of all responders are clearly delineated and predefined in an ICS, heterogeneous groups can operate together more easily.
- The ICS eliminates the need to develop a unique command and organizational structure for each situation, saving valuable time during a disaster.

Advantages of ICS

- Safe and effective response
- Shared focus on common objectives
- Defined and delineated roles and responsibilities
- Preestablished command and organizational structure

- Medical and public health responders, often tasked with working independently, can implement the principles of ICS management to better integrate their response with other agencies during a disaster.
- The ICS effectively integrates the medical response within the overall incident response.

Characteristics of the ICS

Jurisdictional authority is usually not a problem in an incident with a single focus (**single command**). However, the situation can become more complicated when several jurisdictions are involved or when multiple agencies within a single jurisdiction have authority over various aspects of the incident. When different agencies' capabilities and responsibilities overlap, the ICS employs a **unified command** approach, which brings representatives of different agencies together to work on one plan and ensures that all actions are fully coordinated.

Although the term **unity of command** sounds similar to *unified command*, it is a different management concept employed by the ICS. Unity of command means that each person has only one direct supervisor. This concept promotes accountability and may reduce delays in solving problems.

An **incident action plan (IAP)** is an oral or written plan containing the general objectives that reflect the overall strategy for managing an incident. When adhering to the ICS, everyone involved in the incident must understand their specific roles and how they fit into the overall plan. Different organizational components may perform different functions, but all their efforts contribute to the same overarching goals and objectives. Everything that occurs is coordinated within the overall response. In most incidents, the IAP is relatively simple and can be expressed in a few words or phrases. However, the IAP for a large-scale incident can be a lengthy document that is regularly updated and used for daily briefings.

The ICS is intended to be an all-hazards system that can be applied to manage resources at any incident, including fires, floods, tornadoes, plane crashes, earthquakes, hazardous materials incidents, active shooter/hostile events (ASHE), public health emergencies, explosions, or any other type of emergency situation.

The ICS promotes the use of common terminology within an organization and among all agencies involved in emergency incidents. Common terminology means that each word has a single definition, thus avoiding the confusion that may arise from agency-specific jargon. For example, EMS agencies and fire services have used "10-codes" to keep radio communications brief; however, a particular code could have an entirely different meaning from one agency to another. Few agencies still use 10-codes for this reason. By using plain English and common terminology, the ICS ensures that everyone uses the same terms to communicate the same thoughts.

The term **integrated communications** refers to the use of a shared communications plan and interoperable systems to ensure that everyone at an emergency scene can communicate with one another. The ICS supports communication up and down the chain of command at every level. A message must be able to move efficiently through the system from command down to the lowest level, from subordinate to supervisor, from a member of one agency to a member of a different agency, and so forth.

The ICS can and should be used for both everyday operations and major incidents. Regular use of the system ensures familiarity with standard procedures and terminology, increases the users' confidence in the system, and makes it easier to apply it to larger incidents.

The **span of control** refers to the number of subordinates who report to one supervisor at any level within the organization. The span of control relates to all levels of ICS—from the strategic level to the operational/tactical level and the task level. In most situations, one person can supervise only three to seven people or resources effectively. Because of the dynamic nature of emergency incidents, an individual with command or supervisory responsibilities in an ICS should normally not directly supervise more than five people. The actual span of control depends on the complexity of the incident and the nature of the work being performed. For example, in a complex incident involving hazardous materials, the span of control might be only three; during less intense operations, the span of control could be as high as seven.

The ICS is designed to be flexible, scalable, and modular, ready to be staffed and made operational as needed. Any position can be activated simply by assigning someone to the intended role.

Designated incident facilities are assigned locations where specific functions are always performed. For example, command will always be based at the incident command post. The **staging area**, rehabilitation area, casualty collection point(s), treatment area, base of operations, and helispot (landing zone) are all designated areas where particular functions occur. The facilities required for the specific incident are established according to the specific IAP or a predefined ICS plan.

Resource management entails using a standard system of assigning and tracking the various resources involved in the incident. The resource management system of the ICS ensures the following:

- Resource needs are assessed and planned.
- A designated member/group is in charge of ordering.
- A check-in process is established.
- Resource use is tracked and evaluated.
- A means for determining when resources are no longer required and can be demobilized is available.

Organization of the ICS

The ICS structure identifies a full range of duties, responsibilities, and functions performed during emergencies. Some components are used in almost every incident, whereas others apply to only the largest and most complex situations. The five major components of an ICS organization are command, operations, planning, logistics, and finance/administration (**Figure 2-1**). Each block on the ICS organization chart refers to a functional area or a job description. Positions are staffed as they are needed by the incident commander, who decides which additional components are needed for the given situation.

Establishing an ICS

An ICS must be established early, preferably upon arrival of the first emergency responder to the scene. Establishing command is an important first step for any disaster response, and it can be transitioned to supervising officers as they arrive on scene.

Single vs. Unified Command

On an ICS organization chart, the first component is **command**. Command is the only position that must always be filled for every incident, as having a clearly defined leader has several advantages. Command is established when the first unit arrives on the scene and maintained until the last unit leaves. The command function is structured in one of two ways: single or unified.

Single command is the most traditional command function, leading to the term **incident commander** (**Figure 2-2**). When an incident occurs within a single jurisdiction, and there is no jurisdictional or functional agency overlap, a single incident commander should be identified and designated with overall incident management responsibility by the appropriate jurisdictional authority. This does not mean that other agencies do not respond or do not have a role in supporting the management of the incident.

Single command is best used when a single discipline in a single jurisdiction is responsible for the strategic objectives associated with managing the incident. A single incident command may also be designated in multiagency and multijurisdictional incidents based on mutually agreed upon incident-specific circumstances. A unified command

ICS Organizational Structure

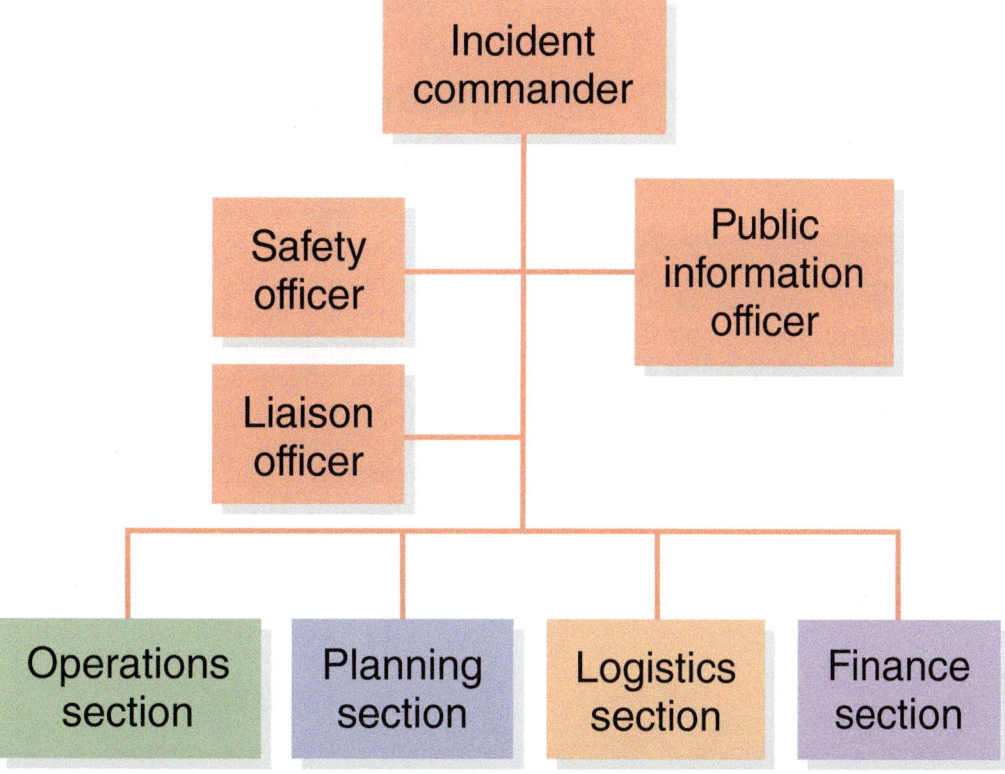

Figure 2-1 The five major components of an ICS organization.
© National Association of Emergency Medical Technicians (NAEMT)

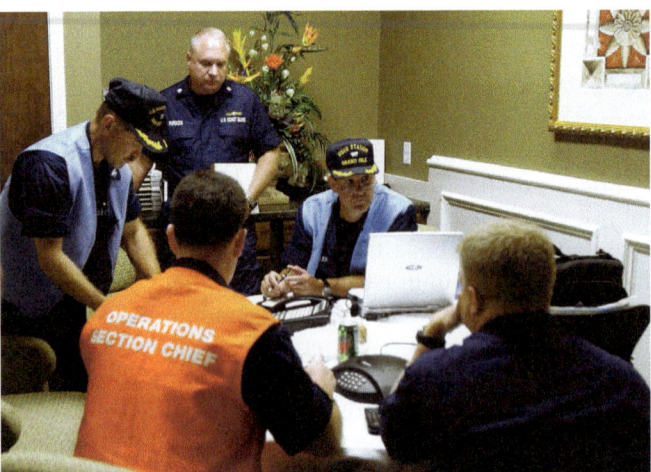

Figure 2-2 Establishing command is an important first step in disaster response.

© Shutterstock

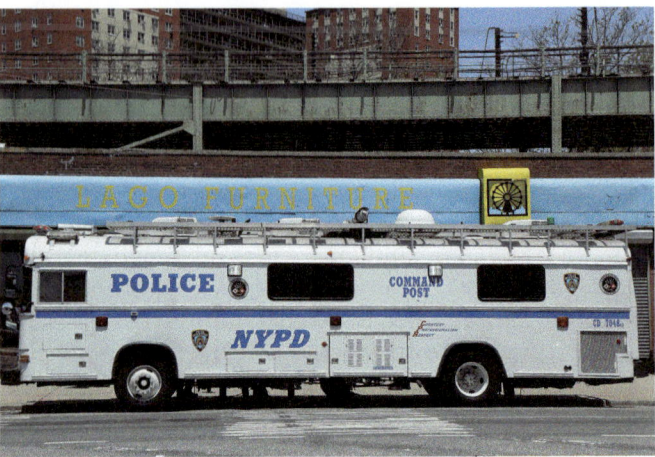

Figure 2-3 For a major incident, the incident command post might be a special vehicle or building.

© Leonard Zhukovsky/Shutterstock

can transition to single command as incidents stabilize over time and their strategic objectives become increasingly focused within a single jurisdiction or discipline.

When multiple agencies with overlapping jurisdictions or legal responsibilities are involved in the same incident, representatives from each agency cooperate to share command authority (unified command). They work together and are directly involved in the decision-making process. Unified command helps ensure cooperation, avoids confusion, and guarantees agreement on goals and objectives. Unified command would be critical in the following situations:

- *Severe weather event such as a hurricane*: In this type of incident, a large number of local, state, and federal agencies are involved and political boundaries have been crossed.

Command Responsibilities

Command (single or unified) is responsible for managing an incident and can direct all activities at the scene. Responsibilities include the following:

- Determining strategy
- Selecting incident tactics
- Setting up the IAP
- Developing the ICS organization
- Managing resources and requesting additional resources
- Coordinating resource activities
- Providing for scene safety
- Releasing information about the incident
- Coordinating with outside agencies

- *Structure fire incident*: EMS is responsible for medical care, the fire department is responsible for fire suppression and rescue, the police department is responsible for area security and evacuation, and public health agencies are responsible for site cleanup.
- *Release of hazardous materials*: The fire department is responsible for fire control, containment of hazardous materials, and rescue; the police department is responsible for evacuation and area security; and public works is responsible for site cleanup.

Incident Command Post

The **incident command post** is the control center for the incident where command and all direct support staff are located (**Figure 2-3**). Representatives from the various responding agencies will usually come together in an incident command post to facilitate interagency communications and decision making and work together to unify the command process. The command post should be near the incident scene in a protected location. The location is often a special vehicle or building on the scene of a major incident. This designated area enables the **command staff** to function without needless distractions or interruptions. For large incidents that are geographically spread out, the command post may be some distance from the emergency incident. The location of the incident command post should be broadcast to all units as soon as the post is established.

Command Staff

Although the incident commander is responsible for the entire incident command organization, the command staff can handle some elements of the incident commander's responsibilities. The safety officer, liaison officer, and public information officer are always part of the command staff and report directly to the incident commander. In addition, aides, assistants, and advisors (including subject-matter experts) may be assigned to work directly for command staff members.

The **safety officer** ensures that safety issues are managed effectively at the incident scene. Responsibilities include identifying and evaluating hazardous conditions, watching out for unsafe practices, and ensuring that safety procedures are followed appropriately. The safety officer is appointed early during an incident. As the incident becomes more complex and the number of resources at the scene increases, additional qualified personnel can be assigned as assistant safety officers.

During an active incident, the incident commander may not have time to meet directly with everyone who comes to the incident command post. The **liaison officer** serves as the command representative in these circumstances, obtaining and providing information or directing people to the proper location or authority. The liaison area should be adjacent to, but not inside, the command post.

At a major incident, communicating with the public and news media is very important for information dissemination. By serving as the contact person for media requests, the **public information officer (PIO)** frees up the incident commander to concentrate on incident management. The PIO is responsible for gathering and releasing incident information to the news media and appropriate agencies. A media area should be established near, but not within, the command post. The information presented to the media by the PIO needs to be approved by the incident commander. Designating a PIO helps ensure that all messages disseminated are consistent and coordinated, which is particularly important during a complex event involving multiple agencies.

ICS Sections and General Staff

When the incident is too large or complex for one person to manage effectively, the incident commander may appoint individuals to oversee parts of the operation. Everything during an emergency can be divided among the major functional components, known as sections, within ICS: operations, planning, logistics, and finance/administration. Depending on the size of the disaster, within each section, the structure may be further broken down into branches, divisions, and then units.

The chiefs of these four sections, collectively known as the **ICS general staff**, report directly to command. Command decides which (if any) of these four positions need to be activated, when to activate them, and who should be placed in each position. The section chiefs on the ICS general staff may run their operations from the main incident command post or from different locations in the case of a large incident, but they are always in direct contact with command.

Operations are conducted in accordance with the IAP. The **operations section** is responsible for managing all actions directly related to mitigating the incident, such as rescuing trapped individuals and treating injured patients. For smaller incidents, command may directly supervise the functions of the operations section. At complex incidents, a separate operations section chief takes on this responsibility, focusing on the tactics that are required to get the job done so that command can focus on overall strategy. In most disaster situations, EMS is part of the operations section.

The **planning section** is responsible for collecting, evaluating, disseminating, and using information relevant to the incident. This section works with preincident plans, building construction drawings, maps, aerial photographs, diagrams, reference materials, and status boards. It is also responsible for developing and updating the IAP. The planning section develops what needs to be done and by whom, and identifies which resources are needed.

Command activates the planning section when information needs to be obtained, managed, and analyzed. Individuals assigned to planning examine the current situation, review available information, predict probable events, and prepare recommendations for strategies and tactics. The planning section also keeps track of resources at large-scale incidents and provides command with regular situation and resource status reports.

The **logistics section** is responsible for providing supplies, services, facilities, and materials during the incident; for example, keeping vehicles fueled, providing meals/hydration for emergency responders, and arranging for specialized equipment. The logistics section chief serves as the supply officer for the incident.

The **finance/administration section** is responsible for the accounting and financial aspects of an incident, as well as any legal/policy/regulatory issues that may arise in its aftermath. This function is not staffed at most smaller incidents because cost and accounting issues are typically addressed after the incident. However, a finance/administration section may be needed at large-scale and long-term incidents that require immediate fiscal management, particularly when outside resources (such as contractors, vendors, and suppliers) must be procured quickly. For example, a finance/administration section may be established during a natural disaster or during a hazardous materials incident where reimbursement may come from the shipper, carrier, chemical manufacturer, or insurance company.

Another example of how this section can be used was seen during the response that most health care agencies launched to address the COVID-19 pandemic. Each individual hospital, nursing home, EMS agency, or other entity that used the NIMS structure likely established a finance/administration section to address the plethora of financial challenges associated with the response, including the need to track expenses for reimbursement from state or federal sources, some of which had not even been defined at the time the finance/administration section was first launched.

Disaster and Specialty Response Teams

During a disaster, a **search-and-rescue** effort is intended to identify and evacuate casualties from the impacted site to a safer location. Depending on the situation, the search-and-rescue effort happens concurrently with EMS operations. The local population near a disaster site, as well as survivors, are often the immediate search-and-rescue resource. Most search-and-rescue teams are volunteer organizations coordinated by emergency management agencies, civil air patrol, sheriff's department, or state police. Generally, they have specialized training in specific environments—wilderness, urban, maritime, confined spaces, mountainous terrain. These teams may have limited medical training (e.g., first aid or wilderness first responder). The Community Emergency Response Teams (CERT) program by Federal Emergency Management Agency (FEMA) provides disaster preparedness training to volunteers.

When a disaster strikes a community, **spontaneous volunteers** often arrive on site ready to help (**Figure 2-4**). These are generally our neighbors and ordinary citizens who may not have the training or experience necessary for the response efforts, or they may be skilled individuals (e.g., former or current military personnel, off-duty responders, nurses, physicians). However, because they are not associated with any part of the existing emergency management response system, their offers of help are often underutilized and even problematic in some cases. At the Boston Marathon bombings, for example, no tracking of volunteers took place; hence, post-bloodborne exposure was not tracked or identified.

A plan for credentialing and identifying volunteers is extremely important because it ensures and validates the identity and attributes (e.g., affiliations, skills, privileges) of professionals or members of response teams through established standards, allowing a community to plan for, request, and have confidence in resources deployed from other jurisdictions for emergency assistance. Credentialing also ensures that personnel resources match

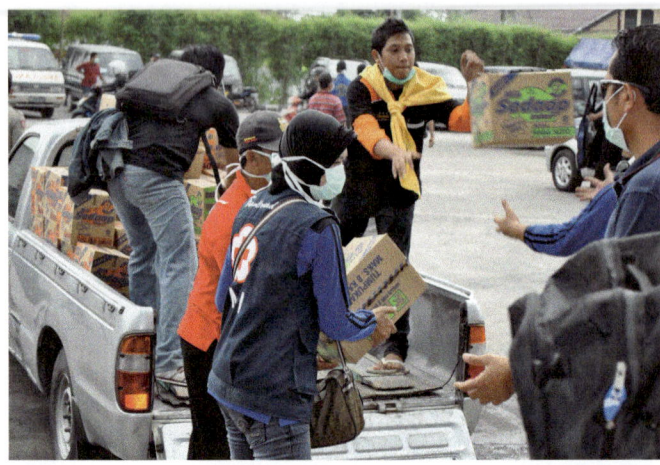

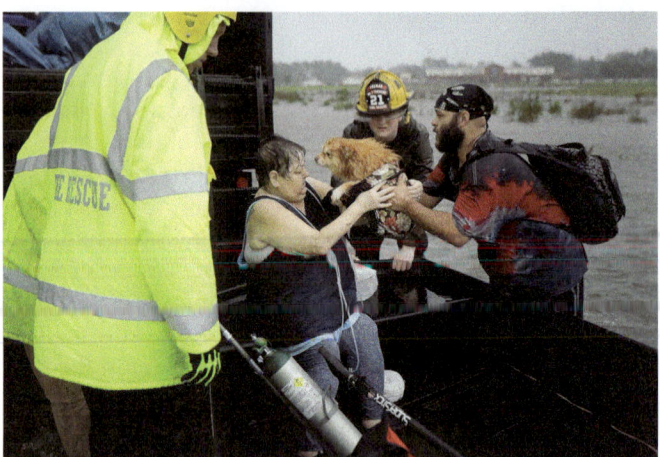

Figure 2-4 Spontaneous volunteers may offer to help at disaster scenes.
© Bedy/Shutterstock; © Chip Somodevilla/Getty Images North America/Getty Images

requests and supports effective management of deployed responders.

Types of Response Teams

EMS practitioners may be part of an **ambulance strike team**. The mission of the ambulance strike team is to provide supplemental medical transportation during large-scale patient movements or other special circumstances. A strike team is assembled at the request of incident command, based on local jurisdiction practice or procedure. Each ambulance strike team has five ambulances under the direction of an ambulance strike team leader (ASTL) in a separate vehicle (**Figure 2-5**). The six vehicles in the strike team (five ambulances plus the ASTL vehicle) must have common communications.

Urban search-and-rescue teams have advanced training in structural collapse rescue, hazardous materials, and rigging and shoring (**Figure 2-6**). They are beneficial in disasters involving the collapse of multiple structures.

Many communities have developed formal, specialized search-and-rescue teams as an integral part of their disaster-response plans. These generally include medical specialists, technical specialists (i.e., individuals knowledgeable in hazardous materials, structural engineering, heavy equipment operation, and technical search-and-rescue methods), and trained canines and their handlers. *Note that activation of specialized teams may take time, and in austere environments, improvisation is often necessary.* For example, at an MCI at a building site, local construction companies may provide valuable search-and-rescue assets, including equipment and tools that can be used to move heavy debris.

Specialized **water rescue teams** may be formed by regions, single agencies, or volunteer groups (**Figure 2-7**). Water rescue teams have personnel with specialized training and equipment that may include small boat operators, rescue swimmers, and swift water rescue technicians. Dive rescue teams include personnel trained in underwater rescue. **Wilderness search-and-rescue teams** are deployed in cases of uncontrolled wildfires, landslides, avalanches, volcanic eruptions, and lost persons (e.g., hikers lost in the woods; **Figure 2-8**). **Maritime search-and-rescue teams** are deployed during hurricanes and in situations involving emergencies offshore (**Figure 2-9**).

Tactical EMS (TEMS) is a specialized role for EMS practitioners that has become increasingly important given the rise in active assailant and complex law enforcement incidents (**Figure 2-10**). TEMS practitioners support high-risk law enforcement tactical units (e.g., SWAT) and train alongside law enforcement officers in drills, communications, and mission planning. TEMS teams may be

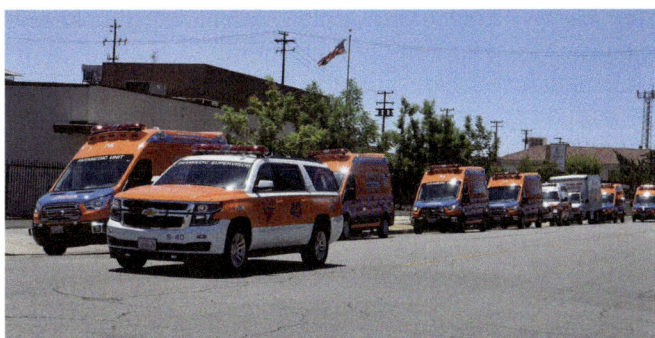

Figure 2-5 An ambulance strike team can provide supplemental medical transport during large-scale patient movements or other special circumstances.

Courtesy of Mark Corum, Hall Ambulance Service, Inc.

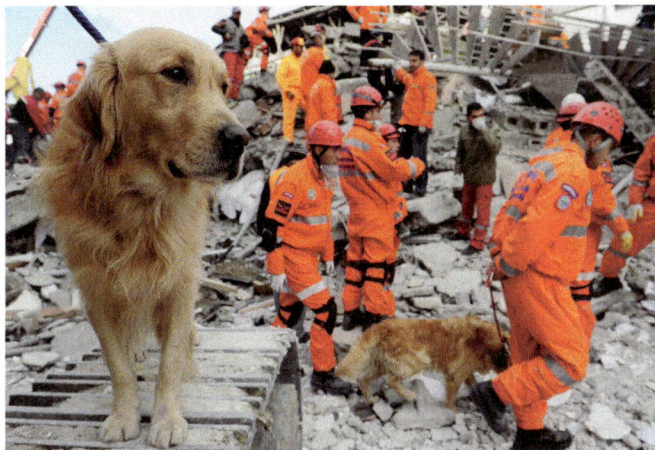

Figure 2-6 Urban search-and-rescue teams have advanced training in structural collapse rescue, hazardous materials, and rigging and shoring.

© 4.murat/Shutterstock

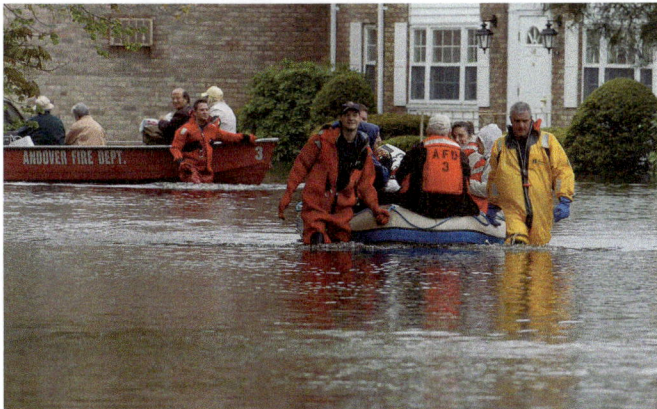

Figure 2-7 Water rescue teams have personnel with specialized training and equipment to respond to coastal flooding and other water-related events.

© CJ Gunther/EPA/Shutterstock

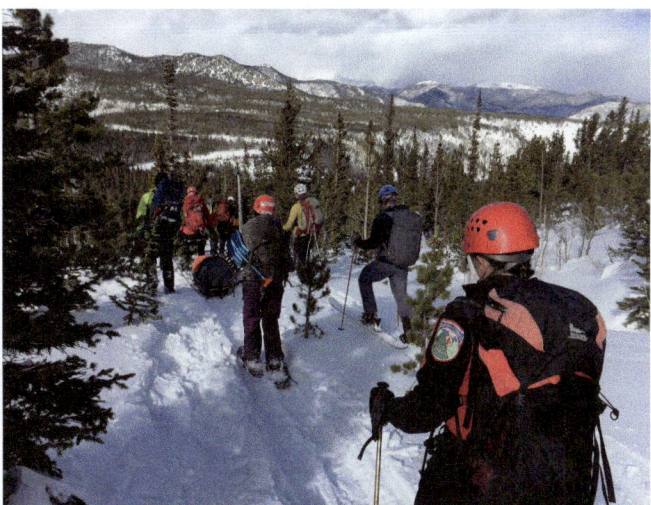

Figure 2-8 Wilderness search-and-rescue teams have personnel with specialized training and equipment to respond to wildfires, landslides, avalanches, volcanic eruptions, and lost persons.

© Rocky Mountain National Park/AP Photo

deployed alongside law enforcement officers during high-risk incidents and may respond by making entry with law enforcement as part of a rescue task force or staging to provide medical support. The scope and composition of TEMS teams varies greatly around the globe, based on the agency and mission being supported. In some cases, TEMS members carry firearms, but many do not. Integrated training among TEMS teams and law enforcement is critical to ensure safety and mission success.

National Disaster Medical System and Disaster Medical Assistance Teams

The U.S. government maintains large-scale disaster medical response capabilities through the National Disaster

Medical System (NDMS) and can mobilize teams of specially trained and equipped personnel to assist with disaster medical response. Some states also have similarly organized and structured teams that can respond to state-wide emergencies. NDMS has several types of deployable disaster response teams, including medical, trauma and critical care, veterinary, mortuary, and victim information center teams. The most ubiquitous of these teams are **disaster medical assistance teams (DMATs)**, which can provide field care as well as augment existing emergency medical facilities when local resources have been overwhelmed (**Figure 2-11**). A request for DMATs must come through the appropriate channels, usually from the local emergency manager to the state emergency management authority and the governor's office to the federal government and the Department of Health and Human Services, which houses the NDMS's response program.

The **National Urban Search & Rescue (US&R) Response System** is a framework for organizing advanced technical rescue teams at the federal, state, and local levels that the Federal Emergency Management Agency (FEMA) may then deploy as part of an integrated federal disaster response. The system's 28 US&R task forces are equipped and prepared to deploy within 6 hours as a component of various response models.

A US&R task force can be deployed to aid in structural collapse rescue and other complex rescue situations. They may also be prepositioned along with other federal responders when the need for federal support is anticipated prior to an event such as a hurricane, thereby expediting emergency response. Following a disaster, the local emergency manager may request assistance from the state or territory, who may in turn (if response requirements are beyond their capabilities) request federal assistance.

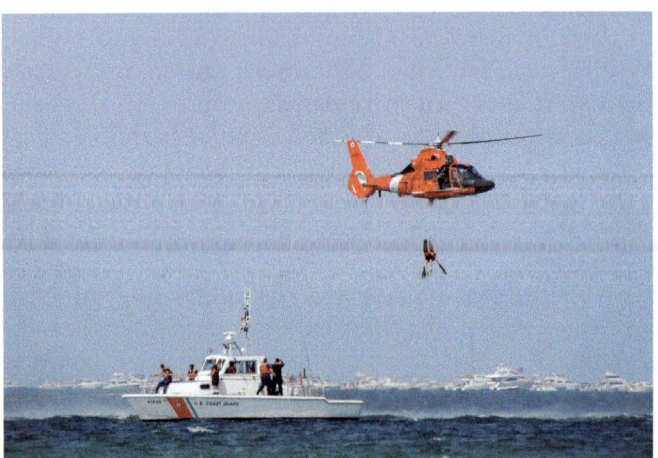

Figure 2-9 Maritime search-and-rescue teams are deployed during hurricanes and in situations involving capsized boats.
© Ivan Cholakov/Shutterstock

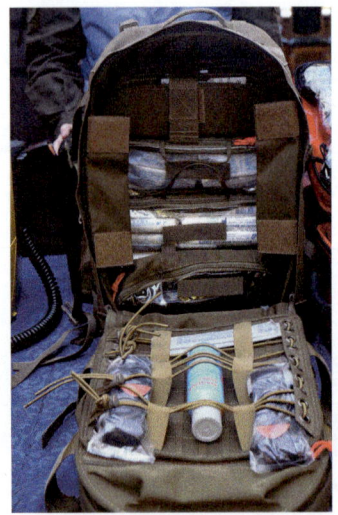
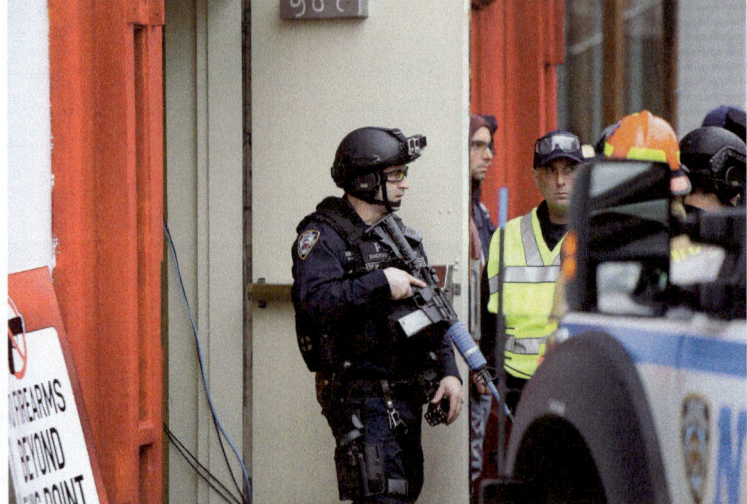

Figure 2-10 Tactical EMS is a specialized EMS role that may involve supporting law enforcement.
© Krysja/Shutterstock; © a katz/Shutterstock

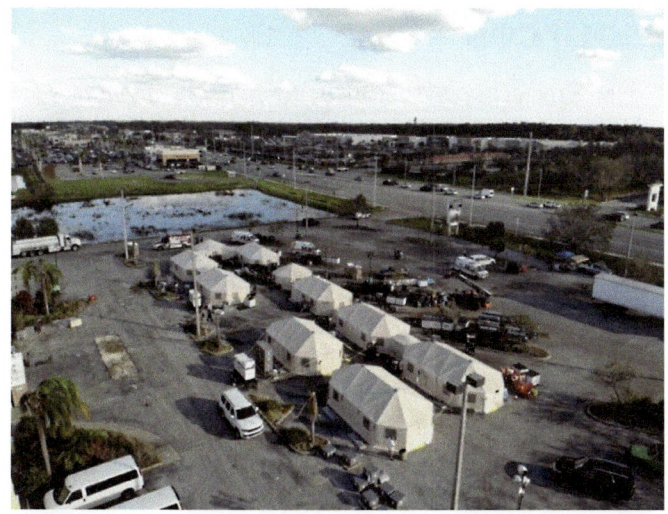

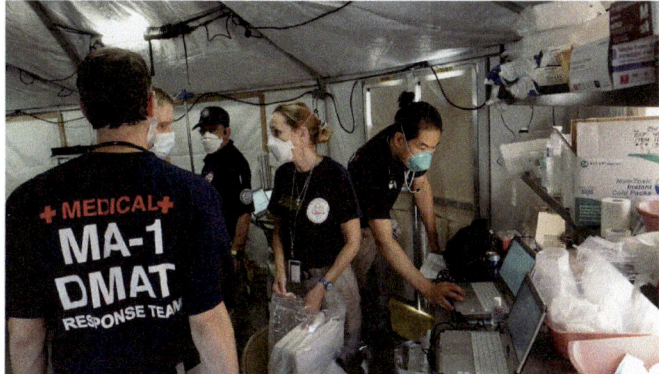

Figure 2-11 Disaster medical assistance teams (DMATs) can be mobilized for large-scale disasters to provide field care and create mobile medical facilities.

Courtesy of Administration for Strategic Preparedness and Response/U.S. Department of Health and Human Services

Managing and Preserving Resources

Care is provided on a spectrum. **Conventional care** is the first and best option. **Contingency care**, which is functionally equivalent care (e.g., using a different medicine to accomplish the same goal), is the next best. **Crisis care** occurs when resource shortfalls cannot be addressed without the risk of poor outcomes for individual patients. It occurs when a sudden increase in demand forces EMS clinicians to ration or triage care. These situations are resolved as additional resources become available or patients are moved to another facility with capacity (e.g., after an MCI). Crisis care conditions may be avoided by acquiring enough resources, adapting resources, or moving patients to facilities with more resources.

Crisis standards of care (CSC) represent a substantial change in usual health care operations and the level of care that can be delivered. This shift occurs when a disaster causes a sustained resource shortage that requires a region to compromise how health care is delivered, putting the provider or patient at risk of a poor outcome. When there is a governmental declaration of CSC for a given period, certain legal/regulatory powers and protections for health care providers help allow for the allocation and use of limited or scarce resources and the implementation of alternate care facilities. CSC should not be considered an option or a choice; it should occur only out of necessity. CSC situations require proactive guidance and a structured response to avoid ad hoc and imbalanced rationing decisions. CSC decisions consider the community's, not just the individual's, needs (i.e., the "greatest good for the greatest number").

SUMMARY

- ICS provides an organizational structure for coordinating emergency (and disaster) response activities.
- The five major components of an ICS organization are command (safety, information, and liaison), operations, planning, logistics, and finance/administration.
- Characteristics of the ICS include the following:
  - Single or unified command
  - Unity of command
  - An IAP
  - An all-risks, all-hazards system
  - Use of common terminology
  - Integrated communications
  - Everyday applicability
  - Span of control
  - Modular organization
  - Designated incident facilities
  - Resource management
- Crisis care conditions may be avoided by acquiring enough resources, adapting resources, or moving patients to facilities with more resources.

References and Additional Resources

ASPR TRACIE. Crisis standard of care brief: Healthcare providers. Published April 2022. https://files.asprtracie.hhs.gov/documents/aspr-tracie-csc-brief-healthcare-providers.pdf. Accessed August 28, 2023.

Federal Emergency Management Agency. Community Emergency Response Team (CERT). https://www.fema.gov/emergency-managers/individuals-communities/preparedness-activities-webinars/community-emergency-response-team. Accessed December 6, 2023.

Federal Emergency Management Agency. ICS resource center. http://training.fema.gov/EMIWeb/IS/ICSResource/index.htm. Accessed August 28, 2023.

Federal Emergency Management Agency. *National Incident Management System*. 3rd ed. Washington, DC; October 2017. https://www.fema.gov/sites/default/files/2020-07/fema_nims_doctrine-2017.pdf. Accessed April 18, 2023.

Federal Emergency Management Agency. ICS Organizational Structure and Elements. https://training.fema.gov/emiweb/is/icsresource/assets/ics%20organizational%20structure%20and%20elements.pdf. Accessed July 24, 2023.

Federal Emergency Management Agency. Urban Search & Rescue. https://www.fema.gov/emergency-managers/national-preparedness/frameworks/urban-search-rescue#Snippet Tab. Accessed April 18, 2023.

U.S. Department of Agriculture. ICS 300—Lesson 4: Unified Command. https://www.usda.gov/sites/default/files/documents/ICS300Lesson04.pdf. Accessed August 28, 2023.

U.S. Department of Health and Human Services, Administration for Strategic Preparedness and Response. National Disaster Medical System. https://aspr.hhs.gov/NDMS/Pages/default.aspx. Accessed July 12, 2023.

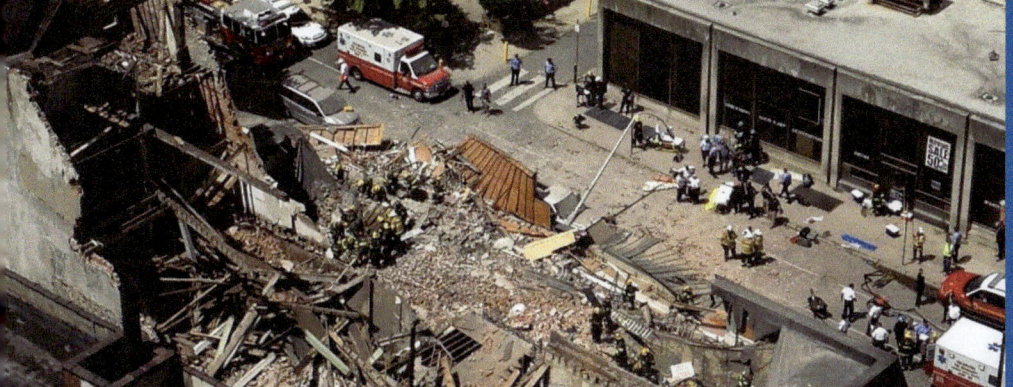

The Role of EMS in Disaster Response

LESSON OBJECTIVES

At the completion of this lesson, you should be able to do the following:

- List the basic steps that EMS follows when responding to disasters.
- Explain the components of an EMS scene assessment during disaster response.
- Describe the main purpose of mass-casualty triage and the various triage strategies.
- List the basic principles of crew resource management (CRM).
- Recognize the factors impacting psychological response to disasters.

Goal of Emergency Medical Response to Disasters

Although the incident command system may address multiple simultaneous goals during a disaster response, the specific components of emergency medical response are aimed at minimizing patient mortality and morbidity. Even in the midst of this challenge, however, EMS must meet the ongoing emergency medical needs of the community not affected by the disaster.

Basic Steps in the Medical Response to Disasters

Basic steps in the medical response to disasters involve initial response, search and rescue, triage and treatment, transport, and retriage. During a disaster, many of these actions will occur concurrently, and EMS has an important role in each of these steps. Overall response may depend on the location of the incident, local protocols, and available resources. The command structure or response framework may vary considerably for international deployments.

Initial Response

The initial response involves notification and activation of EMS, response to the scene, assessment of the situation, communication of the situation and needs, and activation of the medical community.

Notification of the emergency is usually done by witnesses who call 911 (or their local emergency number), thereby activating the EMS response system (**Figure 3-1**). The first units or emergency responders to arrive at the incident have several important functions to fulfill that will set the stage for the entire EMS response. Counterintuitive to normal operations as an EMS practitioner, at a disaster, these first actions do not include initiating patient care.

The first practitioners to arrive must perform an overall scene assessment. This assessment aims to identify

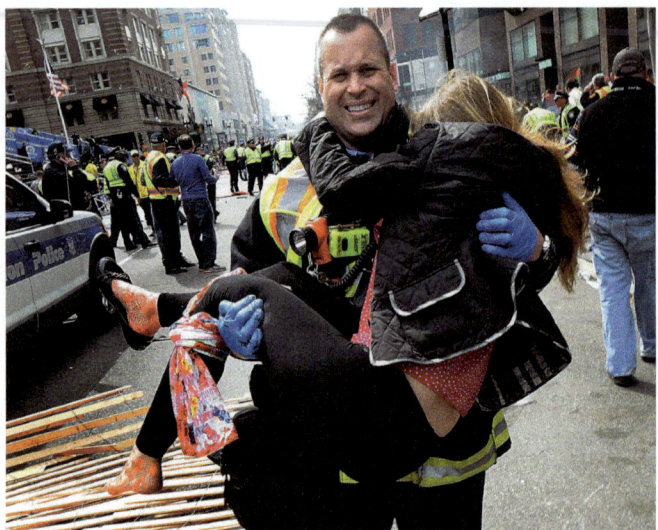

Figure 3-1 The EMS response system is often activated by a witness.

© Ken McGagh/MetroWest Daily News/AP Photo

Scene Size-Up

METHANE

- **M**ass-casualty incident declared by incident command
- **E**xact location
- **T**ype of incident: traffic accident, explosion
- **H**azards present: weather conditions, hazardous materials, downed power lines
- **A**ccess and egress: assessment of primary and secondary routes to scene
- **N**umber of casualties and severity: how many immediate, delayed, minimal, and dead/expectant
- **E**mergency services required: hazardous materials, technical rescue, heating/cooling stations

LCAN Report

LCAN covers the basic information required for a scene size-up and is a simple way to remember the key facts that must be conveyed about an incident. It stands for:

- **L**ocation
- **C**onditions
- **A**ctions
- **N**eeds

---

potential hazards, estimate the total number of casualties, determine the need for additional medical resources on scene, and evaluate the need for specialized equipment or personnel (e.g., search-and-rescue teams, extrication equipment, high-angle rescue). Depending on the incident, practitioners should also maintain situational awareness for potential secondary devices designed to harm emergency responders intentionally.

After completing a basic assessment, practitioners should communicate the information to dispatch through an **LCAN** report or using the **METHANE** acronym. Dispatch will coordinate the initial response. It is also essential to notify the likely receiving hospitals to determine their capacity to receive multiple patients and to let them know the estimated number of casualties with respective levels of criticality. This advance notice will help the receiving hospitals prepare and consider activating their internal hospital-specific disaster plans.

Next, practitioners must focus on identifying appropriate locations for triage, casualty collection, and the staging of incoming ambulances, personnel, and supplies. They must keep in mind the importance of rapid, unimpeded (and safe!) access to and egress from the scene.

Best Practices

- First-arriving EMS practitioners should assume command of the incident.
- The initial incident commander remains in charge of the incident until command is transferred or the situation is stabilized and terminated.
- If incident command has been established by a non-EMS practitioner, the first-arriving prehospital practitioner should establish medical command.

Goals of Scene Assessment

- Assess potential hazards, including a secondary device designed to harm emergency responders intentionally.
- Estimate the total number of casualties.
- Determine the need for additional medical resources on scene.
- Evaluate the need for specialized equipment or personnel (e.g., search-and-rescue teams).

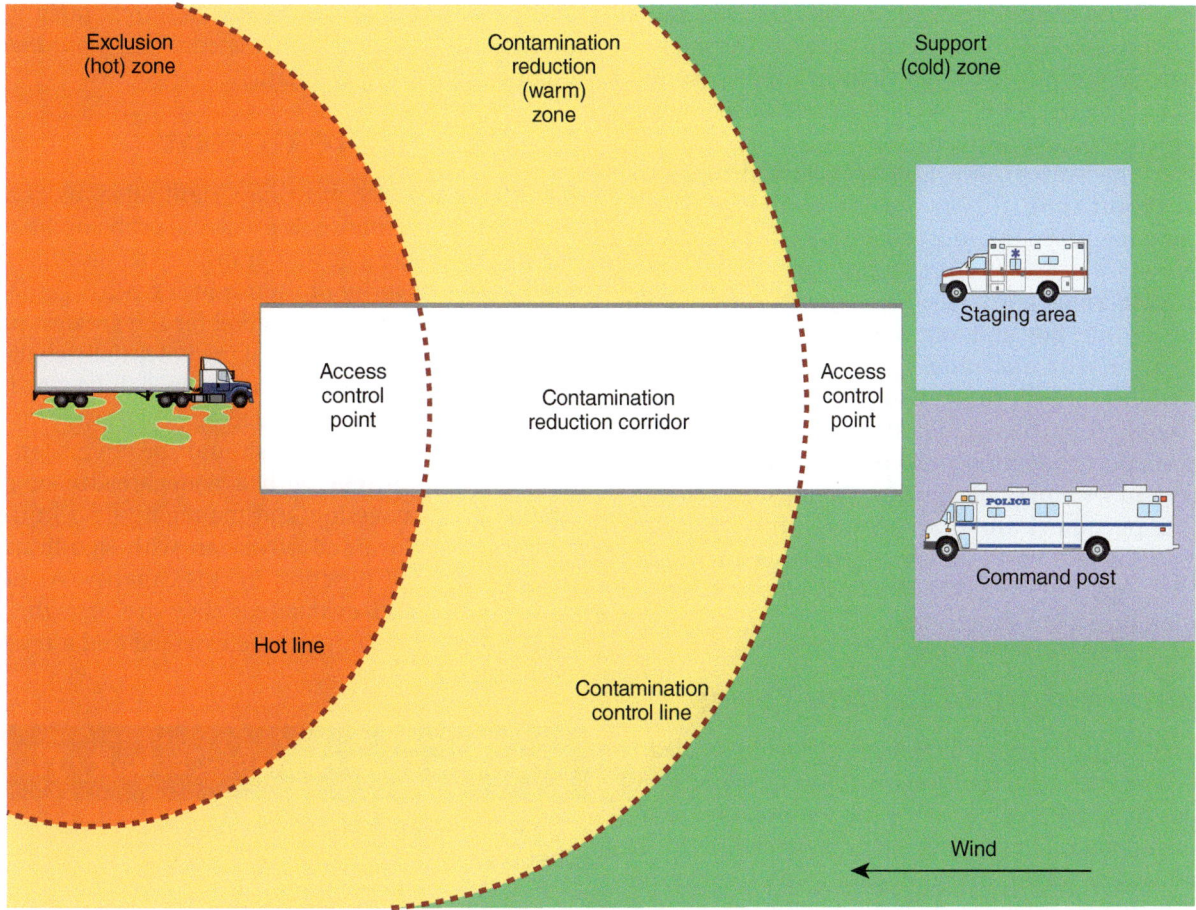

Figure 3-2 The scene of a weapon of mass destruction or hazardous materials incident is generally divided into hot, warm, and cold zones. The command post and staging area should both be located within the cold zone.

© National Association of Emergency Medical Technicians (NAEMT)

Control Zones

To carry out the basic steps in the medical response to disasters, the safety of EMS practitioners is of utmost importance. Proximity to the threat in a disaster is often described in terms of control zones (**Figure 3-2**). These zones must be clearly marked and well circumscribed to prevent further contamination and to establish an organized approach to patient access. Control zones have three components: the hot zone, the warm zone, and the cold zone.

The **hot zone** (also called the **red zone**) is the area where there is an immediate threat to health and life. In active shooter/hostile event (ASHE) situations, the hot zone is sometimes called the **direct threat zone**. The hot zone typically includes an environment contaminated with a hazardous gas, vapor, aerosol, liquid, or powder or with a radiation level of more than 2 milliroentgens per hour (mR/h), or an atmosphere that

poses an immediate danger to life and health (IDLH). Access to this zone is limited to protect rescuers and patients from further exposure or harm. Personal protective equipment (PPE) adequate to protect the emergency responder is determined based on potential routes of exposure to the substance and the likely agent. Level A protection is most often used. In the hot zone, medical care is limited to patient removal/rescue/evacuation, control of life-threatening hemorrhage via tourniquet application, or the administration of chemical antidotes through auto-injectors.

The **warm zone** (also called the **yellow zone**) is an area where the concentration of the offending agent is limited or the radiation level is 2 mR/h. In the case of a scene involving a weapon of mass destruction (WMD), this is the area to which victims are brought from the hot zone and where decontamination takes place. Properly protected EMS practitioners can access this zone for rapid assessment and management of emergent or life-threatening conditions. The practitioners are still at risk for exposure if working in this area, as the agent is carried from the hot zone on victims, other responders, and equipment. PPE is recommended based on potential routes of exposure to the substance. In ASHE situations, the warm zone may be referred to as the **indirect threat zone**. It is an area of relative safety but is not completely secure. Most triage is performed in the warm zone.

The **cold zone** (also called the **green zone**) is the area outside the hot and warm zones that is not contaminated (or with radiation < 2 mR/h). In this area, there is no risk of exposure, and thus no specific level of PPE is required beyond standard universal precautions. This is a support zone for general triage, stabilization, and management of illness or injuries. Patients and uncontaminated personnel are given access to this zone. The incident command post and the staging area are located within the cold zone. The cold zone may also be called an evacuation or patient care zone.

Dynamic Nature of Control Zones

Traditionally, these zones have been depicted as clearly defined concentric circles; however, the designation of the zones must take into account the temperature, wind directions, topography, runoff, spill size, volatility of the material, active threat, and occupancy types surrounding the incident. Products such as the EPA's CAMEO® (Computer-Aided Management of Emergency Operations) application, which uses the ALOHA® and MAR-PLOT® programs, assist incident commanders with the development of the zones.

It is important to note that it is often difficult to define these control zones and that they may be dynamic rather than static. Practitioners should always maintain situational awareness to adjust their response based on the changing nature of the control zones.

Although, in theory, the zones have clear purposes and parameters, the reality is that people and hazards will not always conform to these designs. Factors contributing to the control zones' dynamic nature include the victims' actions/behaviors, EMS practitioners' decisions, and ambient conditions. For example, unless completely incapacitated, contaminated victims might walk toward EMS practitioners in the cold zone or leave the scene completely, either in panic or to seek medical aid at a nearby hospital. Doing so would introduce contamination to the cold zone, essentially making it part of the warm zone, and thus require the establishment of a revised cold zone perimeter.

By design, warm zones and cold zones are designated upwind of the hot zone, but if wind direction changes, practitioners would be at risk of exposure if they were unable to don the proper PPE or to retreat rapidly. These contingencies must be anticipated when planning for or responding to a WMD event.

Triage and Treatment

Triage is one of the most important missions of any disaster medical response. It involves sorting and assigning priority for treatment and transport to disaster victims based on the severity of their injuries. Mass-casualty triage aims to do the greatest good for the greatest number of people, which involves making potentially challenging decisions, such as whether a patient will be classified as critical or as mortally wounded or expectant.

Mass-casualty triage should be overseen by a trained **triage officer** with a wide breadth of clinical experience in assessing and managing field injuries. A paramedic or a trained physician with significant field experience could function in this capacity. As patients are identified and evacuated, they are brought to the triage site, where they can be assessed and a triage category assigned.

The Objective of Mass-Casualty Triage

Do the greatest good for the greatest number of people.

Quote by John Hick

Triage Methodologies

Several different methodologies exist for evaluating and assigning the triage category, including a "sorting scheme" to divide patients into categories based on the need for care and the chance of survival. In 1983, medical personnel from Hoag Memorial Hospital and firefighter–paramedics from the Newport Beach Fire Department created a triage process for emergency medical responders called **Simple Triage and Rapid Treatment (START)** **(Figure 3-3)**. This triage process was designed to identify critically injured patients easily and quickly. START does not establish a medical diagnosis but instead provides a rapid and simple sorting process using three simple assessments to identify those victims most at risk of dying from their injuries. Typically, the process takes 30 to 60 seconds per victim. START requires no tools, specialized medical equipment, or special knowledge.

The first step in START is to direct anyone who can walk to a designated safe area. If the victims can walk and follow commands, their condition is categorized as minor, and they will be further triaged and tagged when more rescuers arrive. This initial sorting leads to a smaller group of presumably more seriously injured victims

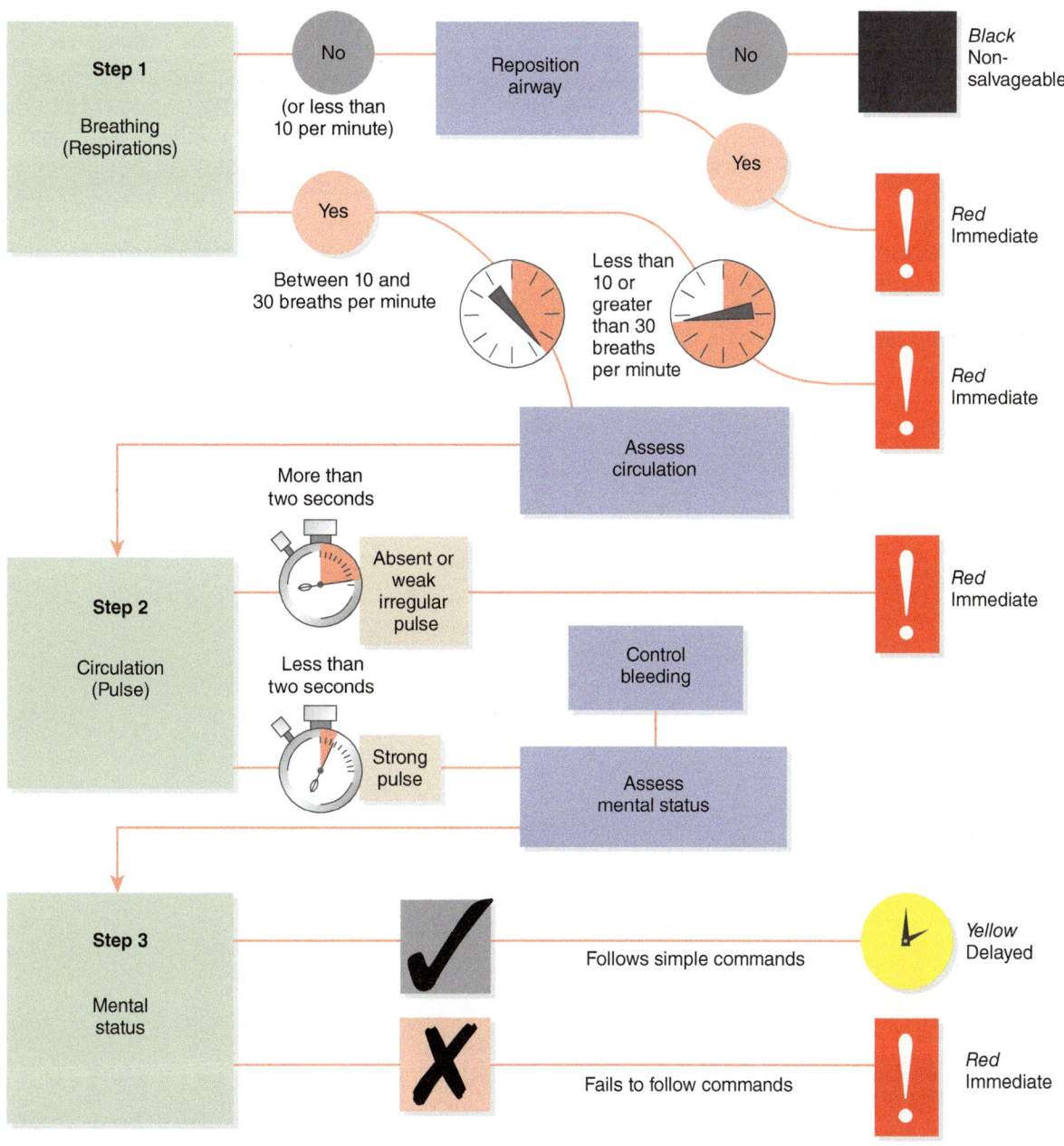

Figure 3-3 START triage algorithm: decision map.
Courtesy of Hoag Hospital Newport Beach and the Newport Beach Fire Department

remaining to triage. The mnemonic "30-2-can do" is used as the START triage prompt (**Figure 3-4**). The "30" refers to the victim's respiratory rate, the "2" refers to capillary refilling time, and the "can do" refers to the victim's ability to follow commands. Any victim with fewer than 30 respirations per minute, capillary refilling time of less than 2 seconds, and the ability to follow verbal commands and to walk is categorized as minor. When victims meet these criteria but cannot walk, they are categorized

as delayed. Victims who are unconscious *or* have rapid breathing, *or* who have delayed capillary refilling time, *or* absent radial pulse are categorized as immediate.

To provide national guidance and bring uniformity to the triage process, the Centers for Disease Control and Prevention (CDC) convened a multidisciplinary group of experts to develop a consensus-based triage system, now known as **SALT triage** (**S**ort, **A**ssess, **L**ifesaving interventions, **T**reatment/**T**ransport). This system begins by using a global sorting process: asking victims to walk or wave (i.e., follow commands). Those victims who do not respond are then assessed for life threats and subsequently categorized into immediate, delayed, minimal, expectant, or dead (**Figure 3-5**).

Like SALT, the European Ten Second Triage (TST) model, geared toward victims with traumatic injuries, allows for rapid identification and basic lifesaving interventions. The TST screens nonwalking casualties for severe bleeding (and allows for immediate treatment with pressure, tourniquet, and/or packing), and then assesses for high-risk injury based on its location to either the chest or abdomen, followed by an assessment of breathing (after opening the airway).

Other triage systems used include the MASS (Move, Assess, Sort, Send), SMART, JumpSTART (pediatric algorithm), and Sacco triage methods. EMS agencies may use any of the triage systems. All practitioners should be able to perform the basic triage functions and be well rehearsed in applying their agency-specific triage algorithm. This knowledge can be invaluable in a disaster.

Respirations	**30**
Perfusion	**2**
Mental status	**CAN DO**

Figure 3-4 START triage algorithm: "30-2-can do."

Courtesy of Hoag Hospital Newport Beach and the Newport Beach Fire Department

Triage Methodologies

- START (**S**imple **T**riage **A**nd **R**apid **T**reatment)
- MASS (**M**ove, **A**ssess, **S**ort, **S**end)
- SMART
- JumpSTART
- Sacco triage
- SALT (**S**ort, **A**ssess, **L**ifesaving interventions, **T**reatment/**T**ransport)
- TST (**T**en **S**econd **T**riage)

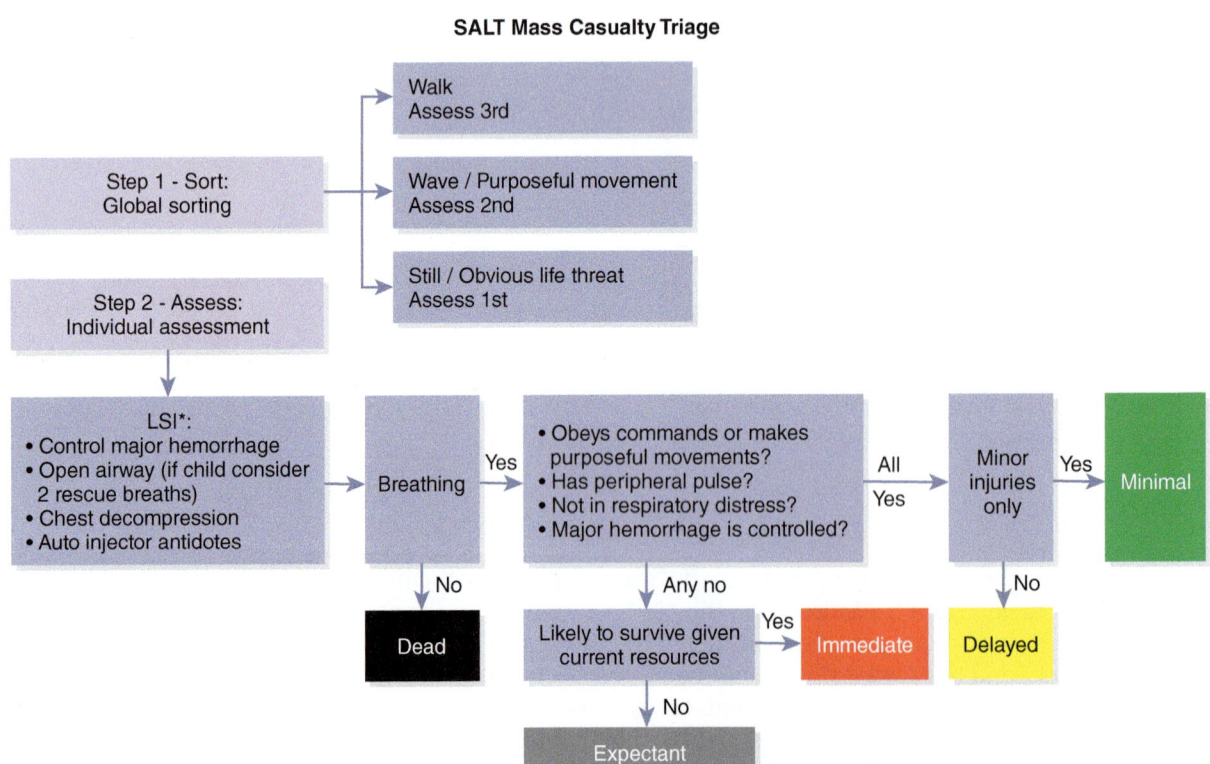

Figure 3-5 SALT triage algorithm.

Modified from Chemical Hazards Emergency Medical Management, U.S. Department of Health and Human Services. SALT mass casualty triage algorithm (sort, assess, lifesaving interventions, treatment/transport). Accessed December 14, 2021. https://chemm.hhs.gov/salttriage.htm

Triage Categories

Regardless of the exact triage method used, all triage systems ultimately classify patients into one of four color-coded injury-severity categories: immediate (red), delayed (yellow), minimal (green), and dead or expectant (black). Some triage systems separate dead victims from expectant victims by using a fifth category for expectant (gray). Triage tags are attached to patients once they have been triaged (**Figure 3-6**). The color code provides an immediate visual reference to the patient's triage category. Depending on the disaster, triage tags might not be filled out during initial triage in the hot/red zone. They are used in the warm/yellow zone.

The highest-priority patients are identified as having critical, but likely survivable, injuries that require minimal time or equipment to manage. These patients are categorized as *immediate* and color-coded *red*. An example is a patient with a compromised airway, significant torso trauma, or massive external hemorrhage. Patients with moderate or debilitating injuries who can potentially tolerate a short delay in care (i.e., do not require immediate management to salvage life or limb) are categorized as *delayed* and color-coded *yellow*. These patients may not be ambulatory. An example is a patient with an isolated long bone fracture. Patients with relatively minor injuries, often called the "walking wounded," are classified as *minimal* and color-coded

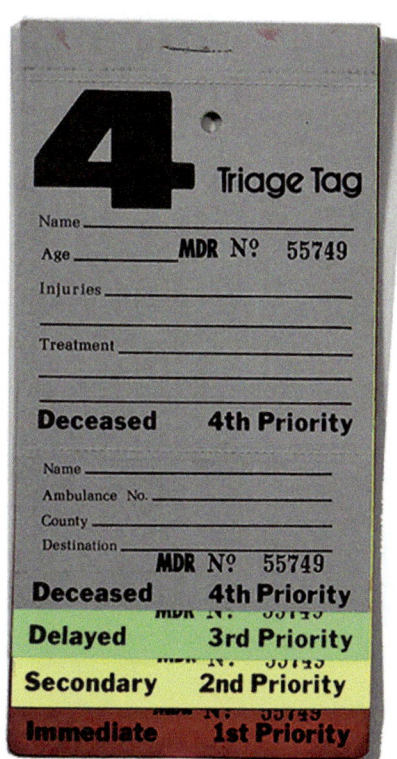
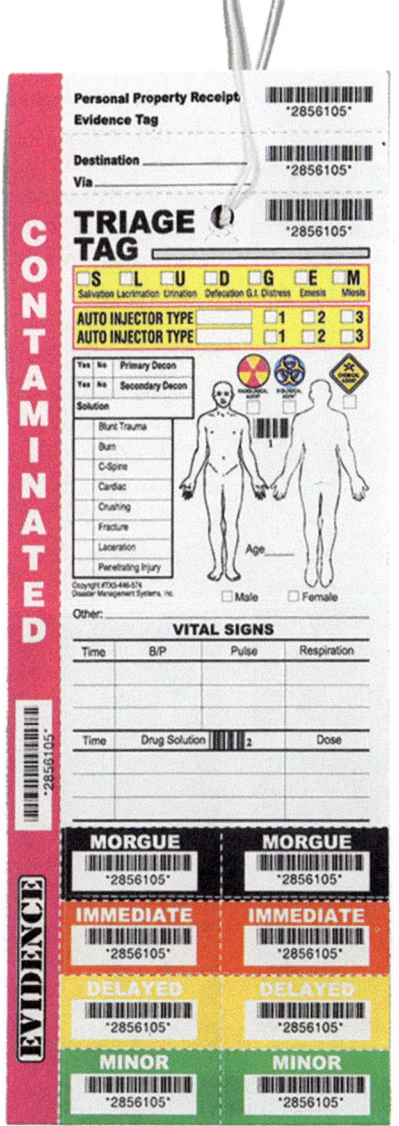
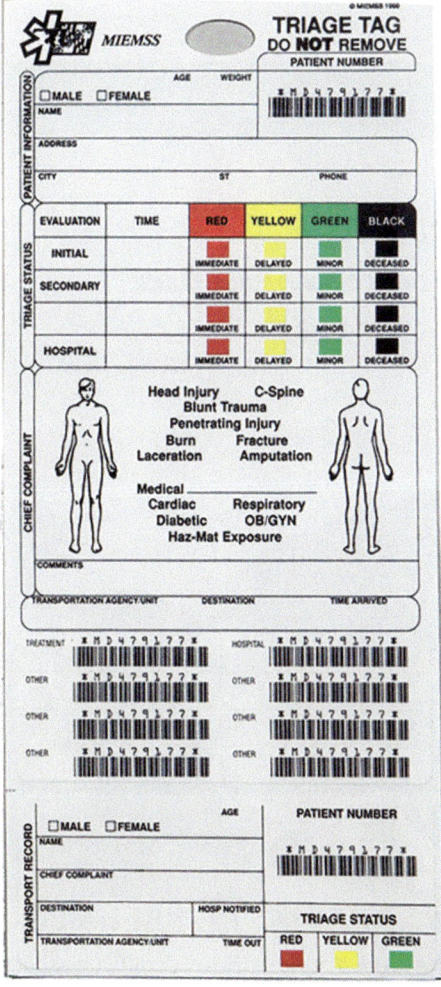

Figure 3-6 Examples of triage tags.
© File of Life Foundation, Inc

green. These patients can wait for treatment and may even assist in the interim by comforting other patients or helping as litter bearers. Patients who have expired on the scene or whose injuries are so severe that death is inevitable are categorized as *dead* or *expectant* and color-coded *black*. An example of an expectant patient is one who has 90% full-thickness burns and thermal pulmonary injury.

As mentioned, some triage systems, particularly SALT, separate patients classified as mortally wounded from those who are dead, color coding the expectant as *gray*. Furthermore, certain response agencies stress the importance of identifying medical (i.e., not trauma) patients by using an *orange* tag. For example, a patient experiencing an exacerbation of COPD following a structural collapse due to inhaled debris may not have a traumatic injury but still requires urgent transport. Because trauma patients may overwhelm trauma-capable facilities, identifying nontrauma conditions allows those patients to be directed to alternative facilities.

Triage Categories

Immediate: red

Delayed: yellow

Minimal: green

Dead or expectant: black

Mortally wounded: gray (SALT)

Medical patients: orange

Procedures Performed During Triage

Triage personnel must avoid the temptation of pausing their triage function and treating a critically injured patient whom they encounter. During the initial triage phase, medical interventions are limited to actions that can be performed easily and rapidly and are not labor intensive. Generally, this means performing only procedures such as controlling life-threatening hemorrhage, providing basic airway intervention, performing chest needle decompression, and administering a chemical agent antidote (**Figure 3-7**).

Casualty Collection Points

Once patients have been triaged, they should be brought to a **casualty collection point** according to their triage priority (**Figure 3-8**). Some incidents will require more than one casualty collection point. These areas should be located close enough to the disaster site that victims can be easily moved and rapidly treated but far enough away to be safe from any ongoing hazard (i.e., in the cold zone). Furthermore, they should be uphill/upwind from contaminated environments, be protected from climatic conditions, have easy visibility and entry/exit routes (evacuation corridors), and be safe from other hazards, such as the exhaust fumes of staging ambulances.

As additional medical staff and resources arrive on the scene, medical care and interventions are provided at casualty collection points according to the triage priority. As transportation resources become available, patients are transported for definitive care according to their triage priority. Necessary medical interventions should be conducted during transport to the definitive care facility.

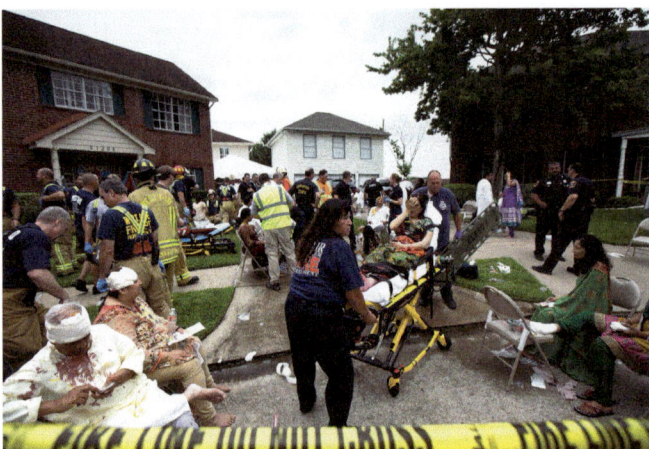

Figure 3-7 One of the most difficult aspects of triage is avoiding the temptation to pause the triage function to treat a critically injured patient.

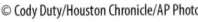

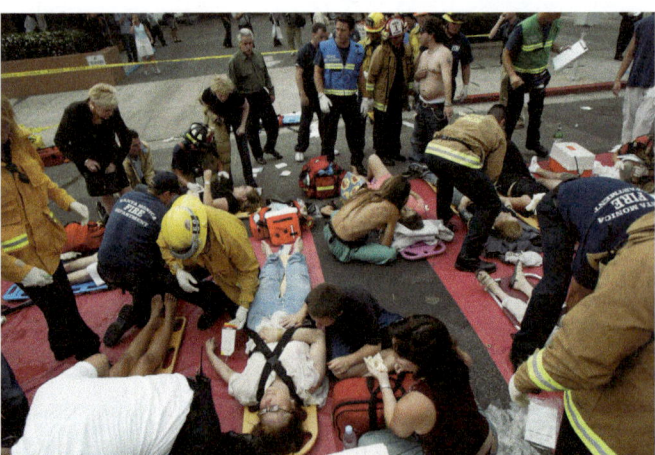

Figure 3-8 After triage, patients are brought to a casualty collection point.

Triage: A Dynamic and Ongoing Process

Triage is a dynamic process; as a patient's condition changes, the triage category may also change. For example, a patient with a major extremity wound and exsanguinating hemorrhage may initially be categorized as immediate, but after hemorrhage control is initiated, the patient may be retriaged as delayed. Alternatively, a patient initially categorized as immediate could deteriorate rapidly and subsequently be retriaged as expectant.

Transport

The act of transporting and tracking patients from a disaster scene to the receiving hospitals involves a coordinated effort using a variety of transport vehicles.

Immediate and delayed patients will be taken to definitive care in ambulances or helicopters (if available and conditions permit). Those incidents that result in large numbers of patients, particularly patients in the minimal category, may be more easily and expeditiously managed using nonmedical transport resources such as buses, vans, pickup trucks, and boats.

When nontraditional transport mechanisms are used, EMS practitioners with adequate supplies and equipment must be assigned to accompany the casualties in that vehicle. Each patient's movement and destination should be accurately recorded on a patient tracking log or via commercially available tracking systems.

Patient/Transport Destination

Once transport is initiated, patient destination is an important issue that needs to be considered. Recent events have demonstrated that patients who can easily move or be moved will often depart the disaster site using any available means of transportation and make their own way to surrounding hospitals. For example, following the 2017 shooting at the Route 91 Harvest music festival in Las Vegas, Nevada, victims used app-based taxi services such as Uber and Lyft. Often this type of self-transport results in large numbers of "walking wounded" arriving at the hospital closest to the disaster site.

Because the hospital closest to a disaster scene may be overwhelmed with patients even before the first transporting ambulance arrives, EMS should ascertain the nearest hospital's ability to accept and treat patients before taking a patient there. If the closest hospital is overwhelmed, EMS may transport patients to more distant facilities when needed. In communities with limited numbers of hospitals, EMS practitioners may have no option but to transport patients to the nearest hospital. Specialty receiving facilities, including trauma, burn, and reimplantation centers, should also be considered if the patient's condition warrants.

Retriage

As mentioned, a patient's status may change during the disaster response. Retriage should occur on the scene while patients are waiting for transport resources. In addition, patients will undergo retriage upon arrival at the receiving destination and again as they are prioritized for emergent surgery.

EMS Safety Principles in Disaster Response

A core element of scene safety in disaster management is situational awareness, and employing the principles of crew resource management is critical in establishing and maintaining it.

Situational Awareness

Situational awareness involves constant vigilance, in other words paying close and full attention to potential threats and all aspects of the surrounding environment, continuously monitoring the situation for changes, and making good decisions in response to what is observed or sensed. It is an active and ongoing internal process. EMS practitioners must maintain a high level of situational awareness through observation and perpetual alertness, communication, and recognition of perception versus reality.

Loss of situational awareness can lead to errors, injuries, death, and delays in patient care and can otherwise detract from the overall mission. The following issues can result in a loss of situational awareness.

- *Ambiguity*: When an action, statement, or comment is too vague and can be understood in multiple ways.
- *Fixation*: A preoccupation with only one aspect of the response.
- *Distraction*: Distraction interferes with concentration or takes a person's attention away from the task at hand.
- *Overload*: When someone has more work than they can complete, more responsibilities than they can manage, or more stress than they can absorb or process, they may fail to focus on the most essential matters.
- *Complacency*: A false sense of comfort or security can cause people to let their guard down.

- *Improper procedures*: Standard policies and procedures exist to keep everyone safe. Deviations from them, such as taking shortcuts, are called improper procedures.
- *Unresolved discrepancies*: A failure to manage conflicts, within the team or with other teams. Team members must call attention to conflicts so that a shared understanding of the priorities and goals can develop.
- *Loss of mission focus*: Not being focused on the mission objectives leads to everyone being too busy *discussing* decisions as opposed to *making* decisions—a situation sometimes characterized as "no one flying the plane." Every team needs an identified leader who can make decisions.
- *Fatigue*: During disaster response especially, people may become overwhelmed and stretched to the limits of their capacity.

Crew Resource Management

Crew resource management (CRM) is a tool originally instituted by NASA and the airline industry in the 1980s to optimize performance and outcomes by reducing the effect of human error through the use of all available resources. It is a core component of ensuring scene safety. CRM aims to enable high-performance teams, such as ambulance crews, to achieve and maintain collective situational awareness. CRM uses a multilayered approach (or countermeasures) to errors that includes the following priorities:

- Preventing the error from occurring
- Containing an emerging error before it occurs
- Mitigating the consequences of an error that was not detected and stopped in time

  The basic principles of CRM include the following:

- Maintaining team structure and climate
- Applying problem-solving strategies while maintaining situational awareness
- Ensuring effective communication within the team
- Employing a just culture
- Executing plans
- Managing workload

Agencies should employ a just culture and encourage open communication among all team members. A core component of CRM is communication. Within high-performance teams, regular use of CRM to gain a shared understanding continually improves performance. Specifically, when teams practice communication techniques that are designed to share understanding, members have opportunities to build team discipline, broaden the knowledge base of individual team members, and remove boundaries to learning. Additionally, CRM can establish trust and respect within teams, reduce the chance for errors caused by distraction, and encourage collective situational awareness. These are critical aspects of EMS practitioner safety during disaster response.

Psychological Response to Disasters

Everyone who experiences a disaster, either as a victim or as an emergency responder, is affected to some degree. Individual reactions to the experience of a disaster vary greatly.

Factors Impacting Psychological Response to Disasters

Not all disasters have the same level of psychological impact. The degree to which individuals are affected depends on both characteristics of the disaster itself and characteristics of the people and communities involved.

Disaster characteristics that seem to have the greatest impact on mental health include the following:

- Events that occur with little or no warning
- Events that pose a serious threat to personal safety
- Events with potential unknown health effects
- Events of uncertain duration
- Events involving human error or malicious intent
- Events involving symbolism related to the terrorist target
- Events involving children

On a more individual level, factors affecting a person's psychological response include physical and psychological proximity to the event, exposure to gruesome or grotesque situations, diminished health status before or because of the disaster, the magnitude of a loss, and

Factors Affecting Individual Response to Disasters

- Physical and psychological proximity to the event
- Exposure to gruesome or grotesque situations
- Diminished health status before or because of the disaster
- Magnitude of loss
- History of previous trauma

Factors Impacting Collective Response to Trauma

- Degree of community disruption
- Predisaster family and community stability
- Community leadership
- Cultural sensitivity of recovery efforts

history of previous trauma. Factors impacting collective response to trauma include the degree of community disruption, predisaster family and community stability, community leadership, and cultural sensitivity of recovery efforts.

Signs of Psychological Trauma

Common reactions to stressful situations are confusion, shock, fear, anxiety, feelings of hopelessness and helplessness, sleep problems, anger, aggressiveness, grief, withdrawal, and guilt. EMS practitioners are exposed to stressful situations on a daily basis; in a disaster, their stress is compounded by the magnitude and severity of casualties they are expected to manage. Common signs of stress in prehospital practitioners can manifest at the physiologic, emotional, cognitive, and behavioral levels:

- *Physiologic signs*: fatigue (even after rest), nausea, fine motor tremors, tics, paresthesia (tingling/numb sensation), dizziness, gastrointestinal upset, heart palpitations, choking or smothering sensations
- *Emotional signs*: anxiety, irritability, feeling overwhelmed, unrealistic anticipation of harm to self or others, apathy, guilt
- *Cognitive signs*: memory loss, decision-making difficulties, anomia (inability to name common objects or familiar people), concentration problems, reduced attention span, calculation difficulties
- *Behavioral signs:* insomnia, hypervigilance, crying easily, inappropriate humor, ritualistic behavior, avoidance/social isolation

Psychological Response Interventions

Intervention strategies are often used to help prevent and manage stress after an incident. One such strategy is **psychological first aid (PFA)**, which applies the concept of human resilience to reduce stress symptoms and improve recovery after a traumatic event or disaster. PFA focuses on reflective listening, assessment and prioritization of the person's needs, intervention, and disposition. Its goal is to provide a caring, comforting presence; educate the individual regarding common stress reactions; empower the individual by supporting strengths and encouraging their existing coping skills; and connect the person with natural support networks and, when needed, professional services.

Alternative strategies include chaplaincy, peer support, employee-assistance programs, and wellness checks. All of these provide teams with effective tools for immediate intervention in situations where practitioners have psychologically related complaints or are showing signs of distress and are amenable to assistance.

The following on-site interventions can assist in reducing stress:

- Limiting exposure to traumatic stimuli
- Ensuring reasonable operational hours
- Ensuring adequate rest periods

Healthy practices during off hours include the following:

- Maintaining a reasonable diet
- Maintaining a regular exercise program
- Reserving private time
- Speaking with empathetic colleagues
- Monitoring signs of stress

Physical Impact on EMS Practitioners

Disaster response can be emotionally and physically challenging for EMS and other rescue personnel. Practitioners' health history should be evaluated and vital signs assessed before they are allowed to enter staging areas. In events that involve many patients and resources, practitioners often remain at the scene or in transport vehicles for long hours while wearing heavy and constricting protective clothing and can become drained by dehydration, heat or cold exposure, and exhaustion. All prehospital practitioners should receive a medical evaluation and rehydration after the incident or after each shift.

SUMMARY

- The specific components of medical response are aimed at minimizing patient mortality and morbidity while meeting the ongoing emergency medical needs of the community not affected by the disaster.
- Initial response to a disaster involves notification and activation of EMS, EMS response to the scene, assessment of the situation, communication of the situation and needs, and activation of the medical community.
- To carry out the basic steps in the medical response to disasters, the safety of the prehospital practitioners is of utmost importance; where and how EMS practitioners can operate safely is understood in terms of control zones—the hot zone, the warm zone, and the cold zone.
- Mass-casualty triage aims to do the greatest good for the greatest number of people.
- Several methodologies are available for assigning triage: START, MASS, SMART, JumpSTART, Sacco triage, SALT, and TST.
- Triage is a dynamic and ongoing process.
- Retriage occurs on the scene while patients wait for transport resources, upon arrival at the receiving destination, and as patients are prioritized for emergent surgery.
- During the initial triage phase, medical interventions are limited to actions that can be performed easily and rapidly and are not labor intensive. Generally, this means controlling life-threatening hemorrhage, providing basic airway intervention, performing chest needle decompression, and administering a chemical antidote.
- Means of transport used in disaster response include ambulances, helicopters, buses and vans, and nonmedical transport resources (e.g., buses, vans, pickup trucks, boats).
- Choosing the patient destination involves several considerations. Before taking a patient to the closest hospital, EMS should ascertain the hospital's ability to accept and treat additional patients. Specialty receiving facilities, including trauma, burn, and reimplantation centers, should also be considered if the patient's condition warrants.
- Maintaining situational awareness involves paying close attention to potential threats and continuously monitoring the surrounding environment for changes.
- Crew resource management is a core component of ensuring scene safety by achieving and maintaining collective situational awareness.
- All persons who experience a disaster have some level of psychological impact. The degree to which individuals are affected depends on both characteristics of the disaster itself and characteristics of the people and communities involved.
- Common signs of stress in prehospital practitioners can manifest at the physiologic, emotional, cognitive, and behavioral levels.
- Intervention strategies are often used to help prevent and manage stress after an incident. Psychological first aid (PFA), for example, applies the concept of human resilience to reduce stress symptoms and improve recovery after a traumatic event or disaster.

References and Additional Resources

American Psychological Association. What is psychological first aid (PFA)? Published March 2019. https://www.apa.org/practice/programs/dmhi/psychological-first-aid. Accessed May 4, 2023.

Arshad FH, Williams A, Asaeda G, et al. A modified Simple Triage and Rapid Treatment algorithm from the New York City (USA) Fire Department. *Prehosp Disaster Med.* 2015;30(2):1–6.

Bloch YH, Schwartz D, Pinkert M, et al. Distribution of casualties in a mass-casualty incident with three local hospitals in the periphery of a densely populated area: lessons learned from the medical management of a terrorist attack. *Prehosp Disast Med.* 2007;22:186–192.

Burkle FM, Newland C, Orebaugh S, et al. Emergency medicine in the Persian Gulf: part II–triage methodology lessons learned. *Ann Emerg Med.* 1994;23:748–754.

Lerner EB, Schwartz RB, Coule PL, et al. Mass casualty triage: an evaluation of the data and development of a proposed national guideline. *Disaster Med Public Health Prep.* 2008;2(suppl 1):S25–S34.

National Association of Emergency Medical Technicians. *Prehospital Trauma Life Support.* 10th ed. Jones & Bartlett Learning; 2023.

Super G. *START: A Triage Training Module.* Hoag Memorial Hospital Presbyterian; 1984.

Vassallo J, Cowburn P, Park C, et al. Ten Second Triage: a novel and pragmatic approach to major incident triage. *Trauma.* 2023.

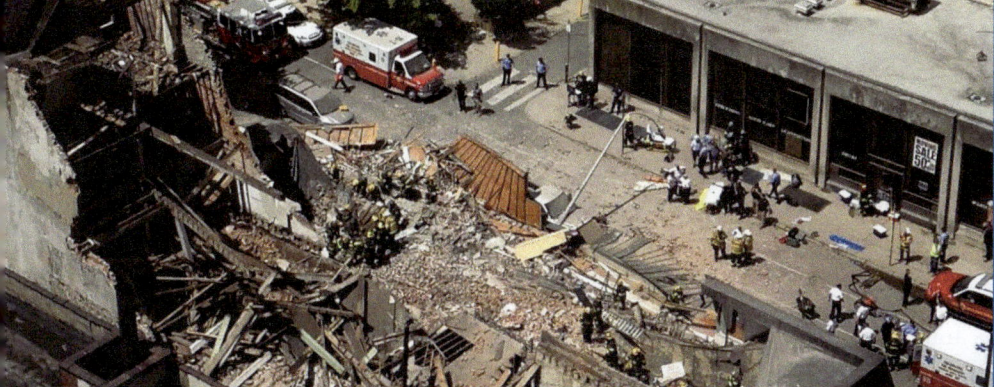

Mass-Casualty Incidents (MCIs)

LESSON OBJECTIVES

At the completion of this lesson, you should be able to do the following:

· List the specific priorities in the management of MCIs.

· State the challenges of MCI response in rural and urban settings.

· Discuss the clinical treatment priorities based on zones of care.

General Considerations

What Is an MCI?

A **mass-casualty incident (MCI)** can be best thought of as a single incident with multiple patients that initially overwhelms the response capabilities of an EMS system. In other words, the number of patients exceeds the available resources, regardless of whether the incident is a motor vehicle collision, building collapse, airplane crash, active shooter, environmental disaster, infectious disease outbreak, biologic disaster, or hazmat disaster. An MCI, whether intentional or unintentional, may have multiple scenes. Note that in some sources, MCI stands for *multiple*-casualty incident and simply denotes an event involving more than one patient.

Examples of unintentional MCIs include the following:

· Building/bridge collapses
· Structural fires
· Plane/helicopter collisions
· Motor vehicle/mass transportation collisions
· Industrial incidents
· Natural disasters

· Biologic disasters/infectious diseases
· Petrochemical explosions

Examples of intentional MCIs include the following:

· Active shooter/hostile events
· Bombings
· Chemical attacks
· Bioterrorism attacks
· Arson
· Vehicle-ramming attacks
· Civil unrest

Key EMS Response Priorities During MCIs

Regardless of the MCI's cause, scope, media coverage, or other factors, the safety of EMS personnel, patients, and bystanders remains the ultimate priority; actions that contribute to additional injuries will only make the situation worse. To stabilize the incident, incident command or an EMS branch of unified command must manage and control the medical response to the MCI. A scene survey is very important to identify the size and complexity of the scene, with additional needs established through the scene size-up and triage findings. EMS practitioners and other emergency practitioners should keep radio traffic to a minimum to avoid confusion but should be sure to notify surrounding hospitals early so that they can prepare for an influx of patients. The ingress and egress routes for emergency vehicles should be preserved to ensure the smooth flow of resources and transportation of patients. Patient tracking is critical in any MCI, along with ensuring continuity of 911 service in the community.

Key EMS Response Priorities During MCIs

- Life safety
- Incident stabilization
- Early requests for additional resources
- Patient triage and identification
- Keeping radio traffic minimal
- Early notification of surrounding hospitals
- Control of ingress and egress routes for emergency vehicles
- Patient tracking
- Continuity of 911 service in the community

Fatality Management: Challenges for EMS

A **mass-fatality incident (MFI)** is a situation in which more fatalities occur than can be managed by local resources. MFIs may be human made, such as hazardous materials releases, transportation accidents, or terrorist attacks, or they may result from natural disasters. There is a thin line between an MCI and an MFI: Whereas an MCI overwhelms emergency resources, an MFI overwhelms resources required to manage the deceased. Proper management of a fatality involves body recovery, handling, identification, transport, tracking, and storage; disposal of human remains and personal effects; certification of the cause of death; and access to mental health services for those affected by the death or event. For example, when a gunman kills five people, it would probably be considered an MCI and not an MFI if it occurs in a major city. That is, additional resources would be needed in responding to the incident, but a major city would likely have the resources to manage this number of fatalities.

As with MCIs, EMS practitioners are under tremendous pressure in MFIs. MFIs, however, have additional challenges. Recovery of the deceased is the first stage in the identification process. There is tremendous pressure from surviving family members, public officials, the

media, and others to rapidly recover and identify the deceased. Family and friends of loved ones may even be on scene. EMS practitioners must be aware of the tasks associated with forensic body recovery and evidence preservation.

EMS practitioners must be prepared to have the scene secured by law enforcement and shield the bodies from view of the public and media. Coordination with the local medical examiner or coroner and respectful handling of the remains are critical. Knowing about temporary morgue facilities, where to obtain body bags, how many body bags your local community has access to, and where can you get an additional supply if needed are all important considerations.

Clinical Issues in MFIs Associated with Biologic Disasters

If disaster-related fatalities are the result of epidemic-causing infections (i.e., Ebola, cholera, typhoid, anthrax), they must be handled with appropriate infection control procedures. Dead bodies may leak body fluids, including feces. Some victims may have chronic blood infections (hepatitis and human immunodeficiency virus [HIV]), tuberculosis, or diarrheal disease. Although most infectious organisms do not survive beyond 48 hours in a dead body, there are some that do: Viable HIV has been found in bodies 6 days postmortem, and the Ebola and Marburg viruses have been known to survive up to 5 days on contaminated surfaces.

EMS practitioners handling human remains have a small risk of hepatitis B and C, HIV, or tuberculosis infection through contact with bodies of infected victims. EMS practitioners should also be cognizant of the hazards posed by highly fragmented remains; for example, body fluids could drip from trees (e.g., after an airline disaster) or soak into surrounding soil, or body fluids could become an inhalation hazard with airborne dust (possible in cases of collapsed buildings).

Patients with Special Needs

Patients with special needs may present various challenges, requiring the practitioner to modify communication, assessment, treatment, and transport actions. Special needs may include a service animal or mobility chair. Patients may use a ventilator, feeding tube, central line, or infusion pump. They may have a vision or hearing impairment or may have mental or physical disabilities.

Caregivers for individuals with special needs will be an important resource when assessing these patients. Consider patients with special needs to be priority patients, to be moved to an appropriate medical destination as soon as the immediate (red tag) patients are transported. Additional EMS practitioners may be required during transport due to the complexity or severity of the patient's condition.

EMS Challenges in Rural Settings

Limited resources leave rural communities vulnerable to disasters and MCIs (**Figure 4-1**). They have a greater need for regional assistance from neighboring communities (mutual aid) and, in many cases, those neighboring communities also have limited resources.

Many rural communities lack local public health systems, so they rely on state public health agencies. Areas that do have local public health departments operate with limited staffing and budgets. Many rural areas do not have access to local hospitals or emergency clinics, and many rural hospitals have resource constraints. For example, some facilities may have limited or no surgical capabilities. Facilities with limited surgical services must focus on "damage control" surgery before transferring the patient to a trauma center.

In some regions, transport to definitive care can take hours and may require additional resources. Inconsistent or incomplete cell phone service in rural areas creates communication challenges.

EMS Challenges in Urban Settings

In urban settings, greater population density leads to higher risks for MCIs and increased casualties (**Figure 4-2**). Although EMS organizations in the urban environment have access to more resources than in rural environments, MCIs occurring in urban settings tend to be larger in scale. Although many urban areas have local public health departments operating at full capacity, departments in some areas may face limited staffing due to workforce shortages. Maintaining a line of communication with local public health and safety departments will assist in the MCI response.

Understanding local trauma center levels and capabilities could improve patient outcomes by ensuring that patients are transported to the most appropriate facilities. However, in urban settings there may be transport complications due to road traffic or other impediments.

Fires, Explosions, and Building Collapses

Explosions can be horrifying and catastrophic events (**Figure 4-3**). During the initial scene size-up at an explosion, prehospital practitioners must gather as much information about the burning substance as possible and determine whether the substance contains hazardous materials. This information is important both for the safety of practitioners and for development of a patient care plan.

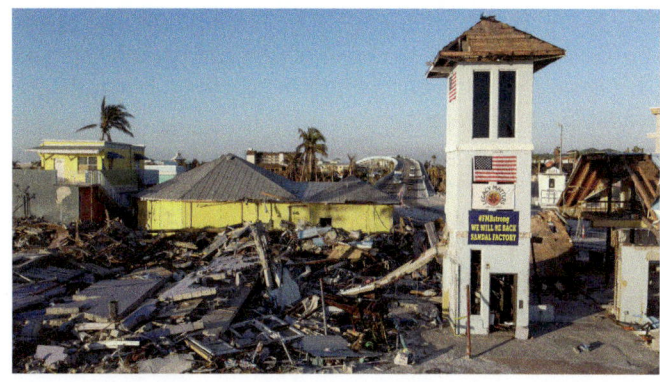

Figure 4-2 In urban settings, the larger population may result in more casualties.

© Gage Goulding/Shutterstock

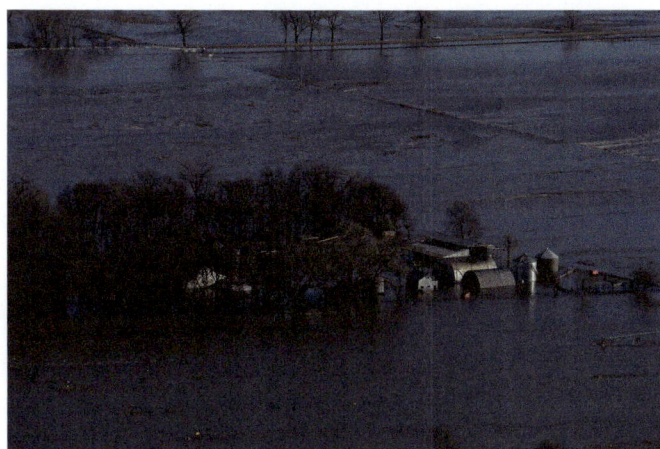

Figure 4-1 Rural communities may have limited resources to respond to a disaster.

Courtesy of U.S. Air Force. Photo taken by Senior Airman Jamie Titus.

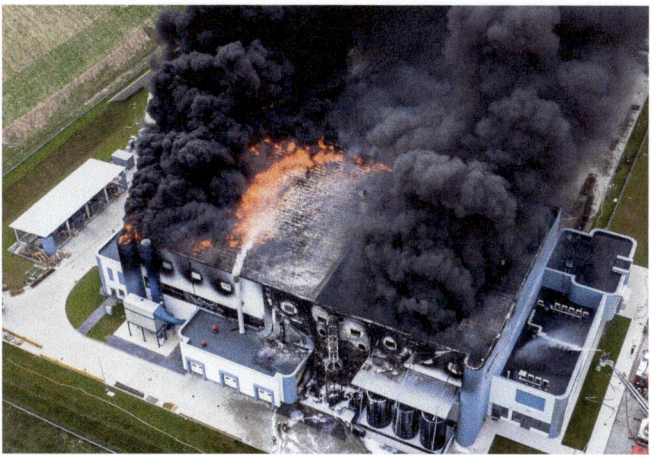

Figure 4-3 Fires and explosions pose many dangers beyond burn injury.

© Lukasz Janyst/Shutterstock

The most common cause of death for a fire victim is not direct complications of any burn wounds, but respiratory failure. Inhalation of toxic fumes is a greater predictor of burn mortality than age of the patient or size of the burn. Because life-threatening complications from smoke inhalation may not manifest for several days, prehospital care practitioners need to consider the possibility of carbon monoxide or hydrogen cyanide poisoning in their patient assessment.

Life-threatening thermal burn injuries involve insult to multiple systems. Heat from a fire can cause airway edema above the vocal cords. Thermal burn patients deteriorate over time, and practitioners need to be vigilant to maintain a patent airway and watch for airway narrowing due to edema. Circumferential burns of the trunk or limbs can produce a life- or limb-threatening condition from the thick, inelastic eschar that is formed. Circumferential burns of the chest can constrict the chest wall to such a degree that the patient is unable to inhale and suffocates. Circumferential burns of the extremities can create a tourniquet-like effect that can render an arm or leg pulseless. Therefore, all circumferential burns should be handled as an emergency, and patients should be transported to a burn center or, if a burn center is not available, to the local trauma center.

Burn patients may have sustained traumatic injuries other than thermal injuries. Burns are obvious and sometimes intimidating injuries, but it is vital to assess for other, less obvious injuries that may be more immediately life threatening than the burns. For example, in an apartment fire, patients may leap from windows or structural elements may have fallen on them. In such instances, the patient will have sustained both burns and associated trauma. The immediate life threat is hemorrhage from the traumatic injury, not the burn.

Prehospital care of a critically burned patient involves decreasing the chance of further tissue damage, maintaining a patent airway, controlling pain, and providing fluid resuscitation. Prehospital practitioners must reassess for any trauma or preexisting medical conditions that may

Fluid Resuscitation in Burn Patients Begins in the Prehospital Setting

Burn patients lose a substantial amount of intravascular fluid owing to obligatory whole-body edema and evaporative losses at the site of the burn. Large amounts of intravenous (IV) fluids must be administered over the course of the first day postburn to prevent a burn patient from going into hypovolemic shock. Inadequate administration of IV fluids may also lead to cardiovascular collapse. Fluid resuscitation begins in the prehospital setting.

- The Parkland formula is often used to guide fluid resuscitation for burns > 15% total body surface area (TBSA) in adults and > 10% TBSA in children:

Fluid required = 4 mL × kg body weight × % TBSA burned (second-degree and higher)

- Administer lactated Ringer's solution or other balanced saline solution:
  - Half the amount in the first 8 hours of the injury
  - The rest over the next 16 hours
  - The goal: urine output > 0.5 mL/kg per hour and systolic blood pressure (SBP) > 90 mm Hg

Transport to a Burn Center

The following types of burns should generally be referred to a qualified burn center (i.e., one approved by the American Burn Association):

- Partial-thickness (second-degree) burns > 10% TBSA
- Burns that involve the face, hands, feet, genitalia, perineum, or major joints
- **Full-thickness (third-degree) burns** in any age group
- Electrical burns, including lightning injury
- Chemical burns
- Inhalation injury
- Burn injury in patients with preexisting medical disorders that could complicate management, prolong recovery, or affect mortality
- Any patients with burns and concomitant trauma (such as fractures) in which the burn injury poses the greater risk of morbidity or mortality
  - If the trauma poses the greater immediate risk, the patient initially may be stabilized in a trauma center before being transferred to a burn unit.
  - Physician judgment is necessary in such situations and should be in concert with the regional medical control plan and triage protocols.
- Burn injury in children if the nearest hospitals do not have qualified personnel or equipment for the care of children
- Burn injury in patients who will require special social, emotional, or long-term rehabilitative intervention

However, in an MCI, you are making transport decisions differently, and the usual transport decisions may not be applicable.

have been missed during initial care. They should consider complications of carbon monoxide and cyanide poisoning and evaluate the administration of a cyanide antidote or hydroxocobalamin if allowed by local protocols.

Transportation MCIs

Many kinds of transportation MCIs are possible (**Figure 4-4**). Motor vehicle crashes (MVCs) can involve both critical and less critical injuries. For instance, a high-speed MVC could have critical injuries and a 1-mile, 100 car pile-up with or without extreme weather conditions could be associated with less critical injuries but an overwhelming number of patients. Other transportation incidents involve bus crashes, train derailments, and airplane crashes. In cases of train derailments and airplane crashes, coordination with state and federal agencies is paramount. Interagency cooperation is critical in managing such incidents.

Emergency medical dispatchers (EMDs) are the first EMS personnel involved in a transportation event. They send out the nearest responders while gathering additional details on the event. In a scenario where a bus carrying people with special needs is involved in the collision, the EMD will attempt to determine what types of special needs exist and what additional resources are required. Patients with special needs may use service animals or have mental or physical disabilities. They could be in wheelchairs or on ventilators.

One regional community resource is a major emergency response vehicle or medical ambulance bus (**Figure 4-5**). The 42-foot unit comes equipped with stretchers to accommodate 24 patients and medical personnel for transport, patient monitoring equipment, metered oxygen, electrical capacity to supply power for necessary medical equipment, and rehabilitation supplies, all in a climate-controlled area.

Scene Safety in MVCs

Transportation incidents increase the risk to EMS practitioners due to distracted drivers. To stay safe on the scene of a vehicle collision, EMS practitioners should wear the following personal protective equipment (PPE) (**Figure 4-6**):

- Turnout gear
- Safety gloves
- Helmet
- Safety goggles
- An American National Standards Institute (ANSI)-approved vest

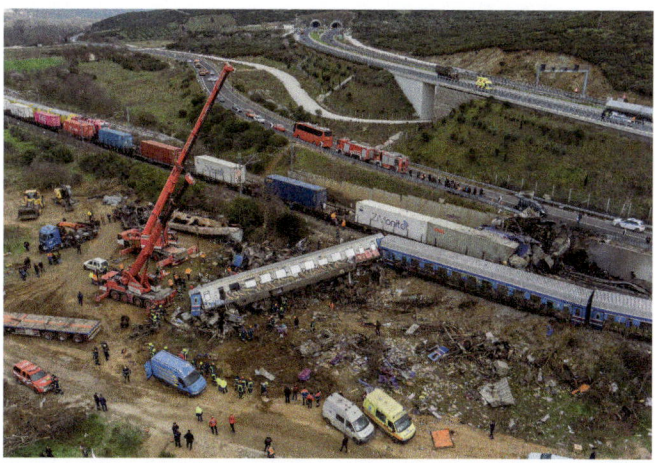
A.

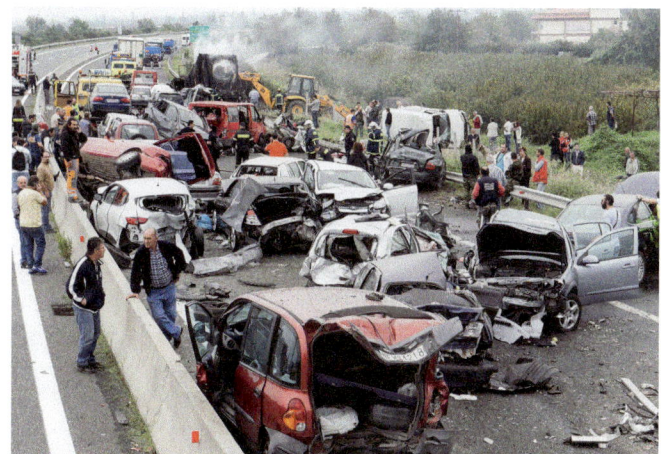
B.

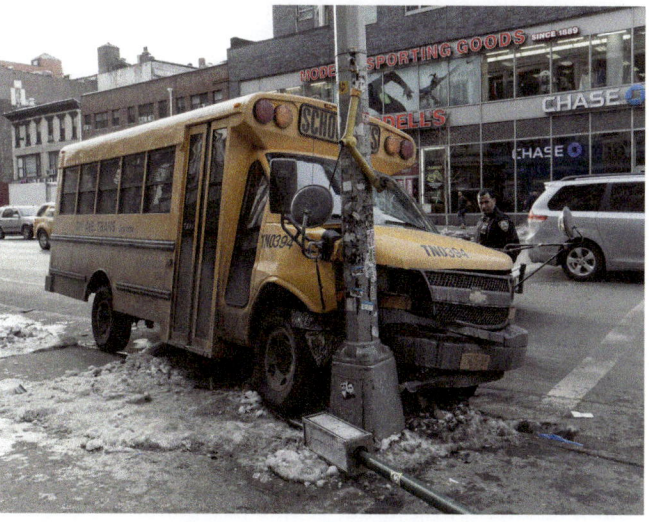
C.

Figure 4-4 Transportation MCIs may involve cars, buses, trains, airplanes, and other forms of transportation.

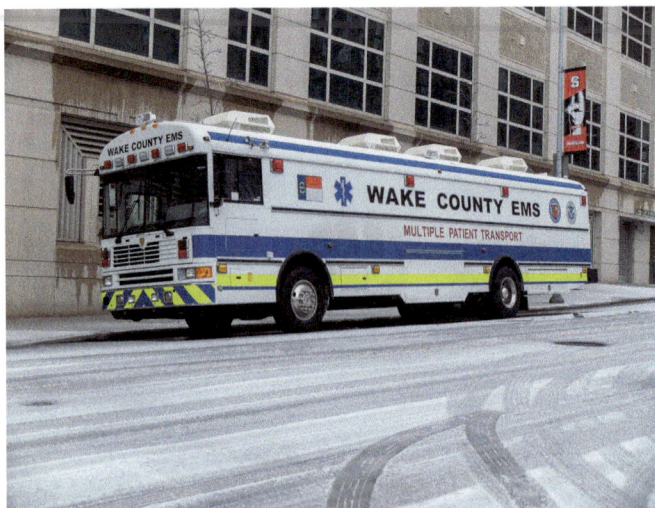

Figure 4-5 A medical ambulance bus.
© Mike Legeros. Used with permission.

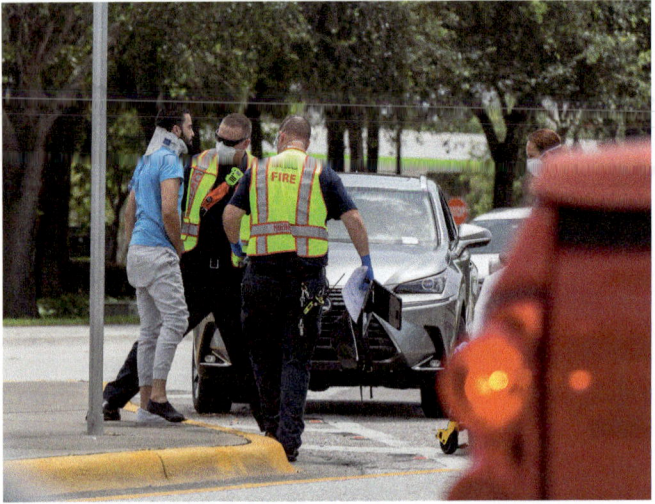

Figure 4-6 Practitioners should wear an ANSI-approved vest at the scene of a vehicle crash.
© YES Market Media/Shutterstock

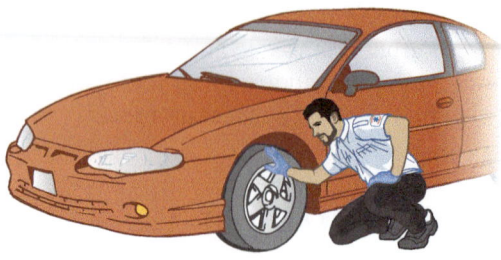

A.

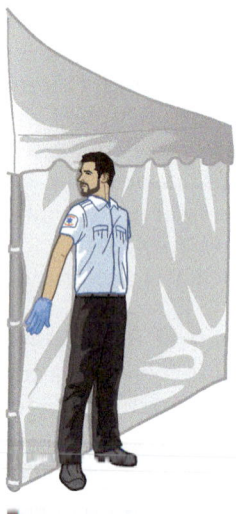

B.

Figure 4-7 **A.** An example of cover. **B.** An example of concealment.
© National Association of Emergency Medical Technicians (NAEMT)

Active Shooter/Hostile Event (ASHE)

Over the years, active assailant incidents have taken many forms. These include active shooter situations, edged-weapon (knife and machete) attacks, and vehicle-ramming attacks.

An **active shooter** is an individual actively engaged in killing or attempting to kill people in a confined space or a populated area. Active shooter incidents are shootings in populated areas that result in a mass killing. The shooter's actions are not the result of another criminal act. The shooter either methodically searches for potential victims or is focused on just injuring people. There may be no pattern or method to the shooter's selection of victims. In the United States, most active assailants use firearms.

Active shooter situations are unpredictable and evolve quickly, as active shooters usually move throughout a building or an area until they are stopped by law enforcement or some other intervention, or they commit suicide. The unfortunate persistence of active shooter incidents supports the need for training and exercises (active shooter drills) for law enforcement, EMS practitioners, first responders, and citizens alike.

Personal Protection of EMS During an ASHE Incident

EMS practitioners responding to ASHE incidents operate in an environment that necessitates specific tactics, techniques, and procedures. Response in these situations includes the use of ballistic vests, heightened situational awareness, and application of important military and law enforcement concepts of force protection, concealment, and cover (**Figure 4-7**).

Force protection refers to actions taken by law enforcement to prevent or mitigate hostile actions against personnel, resources, facilities, and critical infrastructures. Force protection aims to conserve the operational ability of emergency responders. **Cover** refers to a barrier that offers protection from an incoming projectile (e.g., a bullet) by stopping or deflecting it. Examples of cover include bricks, rocks, steel, or a vehicle engine block; however, the type of cover needed depends on the weapon and ammunition used by the assailant. **Concealment** is an area or object that prevents the assailant from seeing a person but does not protect the person from a projectile. Concealment might be found in bushes, in shadows, behind closed blinds or drywall, or even in smoke. Natural terrain offers the potential for either cover (e.g., dirt berm, mature tree) or concealment (e.g., brush, tall grass).

Ballistic Vests

Ballistic vests trap a projectile's kinetic energy and disperse it over a larger surface, ensuring that the projectile does not pierce the body and damage vital organs. However, the wearer of a ballistic vest still feels the blunt force trauma from the projectile. There are five types of ballistic vests based on National Institute of Justice body armor standards. Statistics from the Bulletproof Vest Partnership/Body Armor Safety Initiative indicate that the majority of vests used by first responders are Type II and Type IIIA.

- Type IIA protects against 9-mm and .40-caliber Smith and Wesson bullets.
- Type II protects against 9-mm and .357-caliber Magnum bullets.
- Type IIIA protects against .357 SIG and .44-caliber Magnum bullets.
- Type III protects against rifles, as tested with 7.62-mm full metal jacket bullets.
- Type IV protects against armor-piercing (AP) rifles, as tested with .30-caliber AP bullets.

Basics of Zones of Care

The threat level in ASHE incidents is dynamic in nature and has the potential to change at any time. The type of intervention administered by EMS practitioners and prehospital care practitioners depends on the proximity of the patient to the threat. Rapid changes in conditions and the need to evacuate personnel and patients may interfere with the delivery of interventions.

The hot zone (or direct threat zone) is the operational area with a direct and immediate threat to personal safety or health. The overarching priority in the hot zone is mitigation of the active threat. Medical care is secondary in this zone. The warm zone (or indirect threat zone) is the area with a potential threat to personal safety or health. It typically exists between the hot zones and cold zones and is not a geographic demarcation but rather depends on the evolving situation. Situational awareness is key in the warm zone, and practitioners must recognize that scene security can change instantly. The cold zone is the area surrounding the warm zone. Practitioners can operate without concern of danger or threat to personal safety or health.

Casualties are moved from the warm zone to the cold zone by way of evacuation corridors. An **evacuation corridor** is an area transitioning between the warm and cold zones. It is secured from immediate threat, allowing for a mitigated risk when transporting victims to the triage/treatment area beyond the **outer perimeter**.

A **rescue task force** enables trained and equipped prehospital practitioners, under law enforcement escort when appropriate, to access casualties in the warm zone and expedite lifesaving interventions closer to the point and time of injury. The success of these task forces requires partnership and commitment between agencies well ahead of the incident to ensure that mission objectives are defined, consensus is attained on tactics and movements, procedures are established, and training exercises and drills are conducted together.

Clinical Treatment Priorities: Direct Threat/Hot Zone

In the direct threat (hot) zone, medical priorities are limited to preventing additional injuries, assisting prompt evacuation to the warm zone, controlling life-threatening extremity hemorrhage with commercially available tourniquets, and administering nerve agent antidote kits (NAAKs) in cases of chemical agent exposure. Cardiopulmonary resuscitation (CPR) is not indicated in this environment.

The focus on controlling life-threatening extremity hemorrhage in the hot zone is derived from military experience. A comprehensive study of U.S. combat fatalities from 2001 to 2011 noted that the incidence of treatable exsanguination deaths related to extremity hemorrhage dropped from 7.8% to 2.6% by 2011—a decrease attributed to the implementation of tourniquet use by U.S. forces. To be most effective, the tourniquet must be applied before the victim has lost enough blood to suffer hemorrhagic shock. Despite previous warnings about limb ischemia, there was no preventable loss of limbs resulting from tourniquet ischemia in a case study of 232 patients with tourniquets on 309 extremities.

Clinical Treatment Priorities: Indirect Threat/Warm Zone

The indirect threat (warm) zone requires a focused and deliberate approach to providing patient care. Potential benefits of providing medical care in this zone must outweigh the risks of the ongoing operation and/or delaying the opportunity to evacuate the patient. The goal is for care to occur at or near the point of injury once scene-stabilizing measures have occurred.

Although civilian active shooter scenarios may present similar conditions requiring life-threatening injury management as those seen in combat (i.e., hemorrhage, tension pneumothorax, and airway obstruction), some studies have shown a higher incidence of nonsurvivable head injuries in civilian active shooter incidents than in combat scenarios. Each of the survivable life-threatening conditions is readily treatable with minimal supplies, but these conditions are very time sensitive, and delay in treatment increases the risk of mortality. Because a person can bleed to death from a large arterial wound in 2 to 3 minutes but it may take 4 to 5 minutes to die from a compromised airway, the Committee for

Tactical Emergency Casualty Care (C-TECC) guidelines place control of external hemorrhage ahead of airway control—replacing the traditional ABC mnemonic (for airway, breathing, circulation) with **MARCH** (**M**assive hemorrhage control, **A**irway support, **R**espiratory threats, **C**irculation, **H**ypothermia/**H**ead injury). The principles of the MARCH mnemonic are similar to the XABCDE primary survey.

Massive Hemorrhage

Massive hemorrhage is the greatest threat to life in most trauma patients. Therefore, hemorrhage control is a top priority (**Figure 4-8**). Tourniquets remain the preferred means of hemorrhage control for life-threatening extremity bleeding in this environment. If applied in the hot zone, they should be reassessed once the patient has reached the casualty collection point. Note that tourniquets applied over clothing are not as effective. Other methods of hemorrhage control include deep wound packing with either sterile gauze or hemostatic impregnated gauze. Vascular injuries in the neck, groin, and axilla (i.e., junctional zones) are not amenable to extremity tourniquets. Hemostatic impregnated dressings

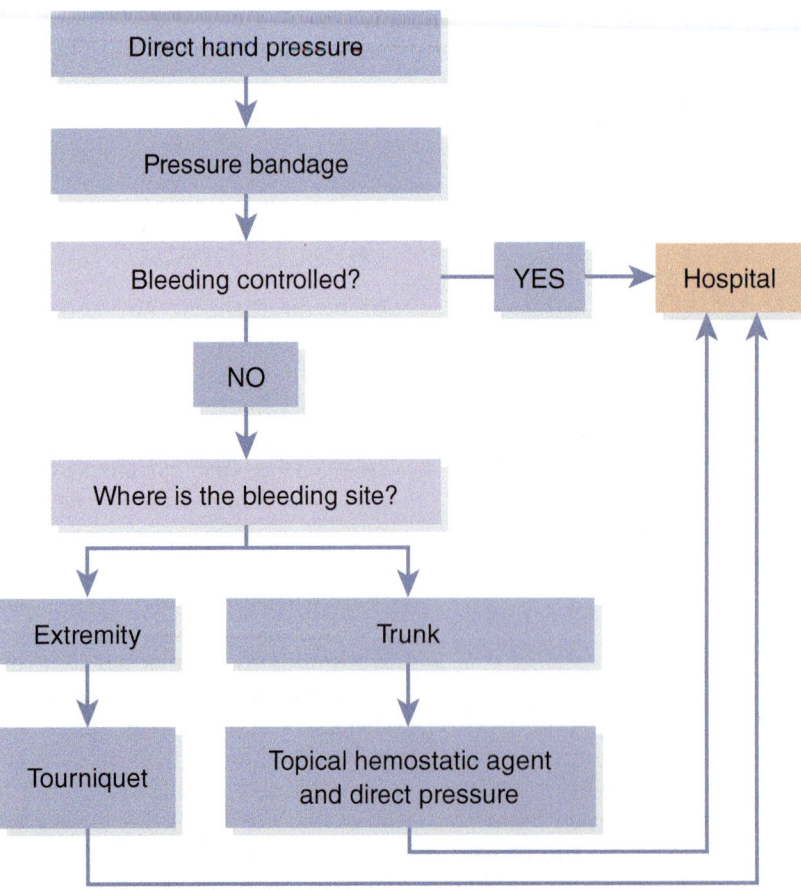

Figure 4-8 Hemorrhage control in the field.
© National Association of Emergency Medical Technicians (NAEMT)

The MARCH and XABCDE Mnemonics

MARCH is an alternative patient assessment acronym similar to XABCDE and used by EMS practitioners working in trauma and tactical situations. MARCH stands for:

M—*Massive hemorrhage*: Control the bleeding of a life-threatening hemorrhage with a tourniquet, pelvic binder, hemostatic dressing, or conventional pressure dressing.

A—*Airway*: Assess for obstruction, and secure the casualty's airway with body positioning, nasopharyngeal airway, advanced airways, or surgical airway.

R—*Respirations*: Assess and treat for penetrating chest wounds, sucking chest wounds, and tension pneumothoraces.

C—*Circulation*: Assess and treat for shock. Establish intravenous or intraosseous access, and initiate fluid resuscitation if medically indicated.

H—*Head/hypothermia*: Prevent secondary brain injury from hypotension, hypoxia, or elevated intracranial pressure (ICP). Protect the casualty from hypothermia. Heat, chemical, or toxic exposures may also be risk factors. Splint any major fracture, and provide spinal motion restriction for patients at risk (from the MARCH PAWS [pain control, antibiotic administration, wound bandaging, splinting] mnemonic).

The MARCH approach aligns closely with the XABCDE approach, which is the patient assessment acronym for trauma patients used by EMS practitioners. A side-by-side comparison shows the following parallel features:

Massive hemorrhage	e**X**sanguinating hemorrhage
Airway	**A**irway
Respirations	**B**reathing
Circulation	**C**irculation
Head/hypothermia	**D**isability Expose/environment

with direct pressure (minimum 5 minutes of continuous pressure being preferred) are effective in such situations.

Airway Management

Patients in the warm zone with airway issues are high priority for evacuation due to intense resource requirements to manage airway trauma. Consider applying oxygen if available and indicated. In patients with airway obstruction, or impending obstruction, apply a chin-lift or jaw-thrust (preferred) maneuver, use a nasopharyngeal airway (if not contraindicated), and place the patient in the position that best protects the airway (sitting up or leaning forward). If the patient is unconscious, then place the patient in the recovery position. If these measures are unsuccessful, consider blind insertion airway devices (BIAD; extraglottic/supraglottic airways) based on protocol. Keep in mind, however, that you may not be able to stay with the patient to continue BVM ventilations.

Respirations

Assess the chest/upper abdomen for any evidence of an open chest wound and apply an occlusive dressing accordingly. Monitor the patient for signs of impending tension pneumothorax (**Figure 4-9**).

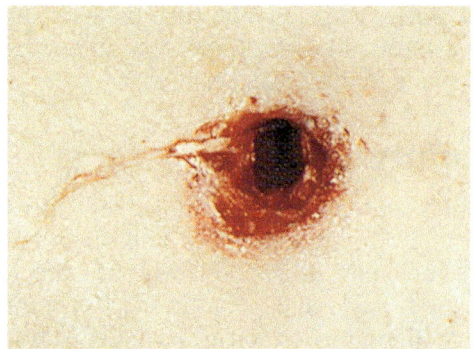

A.

B.

Figure 4-9   A. A gunshot or stab wound to the chest produces a hole in the chest wall through which air can flow both into and out of the pleural cavity. **B.** Vented chest seals have been shown in animal studies to prevent the development of tension pneumothorax.

Circulation

In general, healthy adult trauma patients with a radial pulse and normal mentation do not need IV therapy in the warm zone. In patients with evidence of hypotension and signs of a closed head injury, IV fluid therapy is indicated to maintain at least a radial pulse, or SBP of at least 90 mm Hg (> 110 mm Hg for patients with head trauma). Patients in hypovolemic shock should receive a one-time 500-mL bolus of IV fluid to achieve SBP goals. Patients in traumatic cardiac arrest with evidence of thoracic trauma should receive bilateral needle decompression and reassessment.

Hypothermia

Hypothermia in trauma patients has been associated with increased mortality because cellular functions are affected and clotting is diminished (**Figure 4-10**). Hypothermia is easier to prevent than to treat, and hypothermia prevention is the easiest part of the lethal triad to control. To prevent hypothermia, patients should be moved to a warmed location if possible and other efforts should be made to minimize heat loss.

Head Injury

Identification and appropriate triage of patients with severe head injury is extremely important for better long-term outcomes. In a patient who has altered mental status due to suspected or confirmed severe traumatic brain injury (Glasgow Coma Scale [GCS] < 9), resuscitate with fluid boluses until mental status improves, strong pulses are felt, or SBP is >110 mm Hg, and position the patient with head elevated 30 degrees, if possible, with neck neutral. Avoid an overly tight cervical collar or

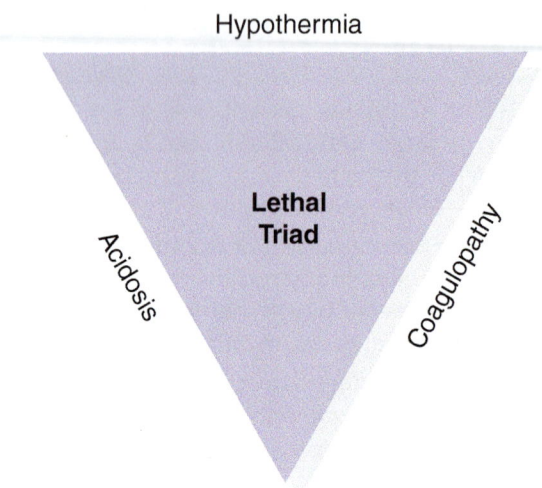

Figure 4-10 Lethal triad.
© Jones & Bartlett Learning

airway securing devices that may impede venous outflow from the head.

Clinical Treatment Priorities: Cold Zone

Casualties will require retriage, particularly assessment of the development of a life-threatening condition and effects of warm zone therapy. Massive hemorrhage should be immediately readdressed. Patients should be triaged and transported per standard practices. Medical care in the cold zone should be dictated by resource availability and, when possible, equate to the general patient care standards. CPR may have a larger role in the cold zone, depending on the available resources.

SUMMARY

- Priorities in an MCI are life safety, incident stabilization, early requests for additional resources, patient triage and identification, considerate use of radio traffic, early notification of surrounding hospitals, control of ingress and egress routes for emergency vehicles, patient tracking, and continuity of 911 service in the community.
- In case of multiple fatalities, EMS practitioners are faced with the challenge of recovery and identification of the deceased and shielding the bodies from the view of the media and public.
- Law enforcement, fire department, and EMS share the same priorities during an MCI; interagency cooperation should be paramount.

- Patients with special needs should be transported after "red-tag" patients.
- In an apartment fire with possible structural collapse, the immediate life threat may be hemorrhage from a traumatic injury, not the burn.
- The prehospital care of a critically burned patient involves decreasing the chance of further tissue damage, maintaining a patent airway, providing pain control, and providing fluid resuscitation.
- EMDs are the first EMS personnel involved in a transportation event.
- To stay safe on the scene of a vehicle collision, EMS practitioners should wear the following PPE: turnout

SUMMARY (CONTINUED)

- gear, safety gloves, helmet, safety goggles, and an ANSI-approved vest.
- EMS practitioners responding to active shooter events operate in an environment that involves different tactics, techniques, and procedures; for example, they will need to wear ballistic vests, ensure heightened situational awareness, and apply concepts such as force protection, concealment, and cover.
- An evacuation corridor is an area transitioning between the warm and cold zones. It is secured from immediate threat, allowing for a mitigated risk when transporting victims from the casualty collection points to the triage/treatment area beyond the outer perimeter.
- A rescue task force enables trained and equipped prehospital practitioners, under law enforcement escort when appropriate, to access casualties in the warm zone and expedite lifesaving interventions closer to the point and time of injury.
- In the hot zone during ASHE incidents, medical priorities are limited to preventing additional injuries, assisting prompt evacuation to the warm zone, controlling life-threatening extremity hemorrhage with commercially available tourniquets, and administering NAAKs.
- In the warm zone in ASHE incidents, treatment priorities follow the MARCH mnemonic: **M**assive hemorrhage control, **A**irway support, **R**espiratory threats, **C**irculation (prevent shock), and **H**ypothermia/**H**ead injury. The principles of the MARCH mnemonic are similar to the XABCDE primary survey approach used by EMS practitioners.
- Medical care in the cold zone should be dictated by resource availability and, when possible, equate to the general patient care standards in ASHE incidents.

References and Additional Resources

Administration for Strategic Preparedness and Response, U.S. Department of Health and Human Services. Topic collection: fatality management. Updated August 28, 2023. https://asprtracie.hhs.gov/technical-resources/65/fatality-management/0#:~:text=Mass%20fatality%20incidents%20are%20defined,considered%20a%20mass%20fatality%20incident. Accessed August 28, 2023.

Aehlert B. *Paramedic Practice Today: Above and Beyond.* (Revised reprint). Jones & Bartlett Learning; 2011.

Altevogt BM, Stroud C, Hanson SL, et al., eds; Institute of Medicine (US) Committee on Guidance for Establishing Standards of Care for Use in Disaster Situations. *Guidance for Establishing Crisis Standards of Care for Use in Disaster Situations: A Letter Report.* National Academies Press; 2009.

American College of Surgeons. *Strategies to Enhance Survival in Active Shooter and Intentional Mass Casualty Events: A Compendium.* Bulletin, 100(15). September 2015. https://www.facs.org/media/0svpk45s/hartford_consensus_compendium.pdf. Accessed June 2, 2023.

American College Committee on Trauma. *Guidelines for the Operations of Burn Units: Resources for Optimal Care of the Injured Patient.* American College of Surgeons; 2006:79–86.

Blair JP, Schweit KW. *A Study of Active Shooter Incidents, 2000–2013.* Texas State University and Federal Bureau of Investigation, U.S. Department of Justice; 2014.

Cordner S, Coninx R, Kim H-J, et al. *Management of Dead Bodies: A Field Manual for First Responders.* 2nd ed. Pan American Health Organization; 2016.

Division of Public Health. (n.d.). *Children with Special Health Care Needs: Provider Manual.* Georgia Department of Public Health. https://dph.georgia.gov/sites/dph.georgia.gov/files/cwshcnprovidermanual.04.pdf. Accessed June 2, 2023.

Emergency Management Institute. *IS-907: Active Shooter; What You Can Do. Student Manual.* National Protection and Programs Directorate/Office of Infrastructure Protection, U.S. Department of Homeland Security; 2015. https://training.fema.gov/is/courseoverview.aspx?code=is-907&lang=en. Accessed June 2, 2023.

Emergency Medical Task Force. *Ambulance Strike Team Standard Operating Guidelines.* Texas Department of Health; 2012. https://cbrac.org/wp-content/uploads/2021/02/ast.pdf. Accessed June 2, 2023.

Federal Emergency Management Agency. *National Incident Management System: Training Program.* U.S. Department of Homeland Security; 2011.

Federal Emergency Management Agency. *National Response Framework.* 2nd ed. U.S. Department of Homeland Security; 2013. https://training.fema.gov/hiedu/highref/national%20response%20framework-second%20ed-may%202013-natresp.pdf. Accessed June 2, 2023.

Federal Emergency Management Agency. *Operational Templates and Guidance for EMS Mass Incident Deployment.* Department of Homeland Security; 2012. https://www.usfa.fema.gov/downloads/pdf/publications/templates_guidance_ems_mass_incident_deployment.pdf. Accessed June 2, 2023.

Federal Highway Administration. *Evacuating Populations with Special Needs: Routes to Effective Evacuation Planning Primer Series.* U.S. Department of Transportation; 2009. https://ops.fhwa.dot.gov/publications/fhwahop09022/. Accessed June 2, 2023.

Hanfling D, Altevogt BM, Viswanathan K, Gostin LO, eds. *Crisis Standards of Care: A Systems Framework for Catastrophic Disaster Response. Volume 1: Introduction and CSC Framework*. Institute of Medicine of the National Academies; 2012.

Institute of Medicine. *Preparedness and Response to a Rural Mass Casualty Incident: Workshop Summary*. National Academies Press; 2011.

Los Angeles County Emergency Medical Services Agency. *Mass Fatality Guide for Healthcare Entities*. Los Angeles County Department of Health Services; 2013.

National Institute of Justice. *Selection and Application Guide to Ballistic-Resistant Body Armor for Law Enforcement, Corrections and Public Safety*. U.S. Department of Justice; 2014. https://www.ncjrs.gov/pdffiles1/nij/247281.pdf. Accessed June 2, 2023.

NC EMSC Advisory Committee. *Recommended EMS Guidelines for Children and Youth With Special Health Care Needs (CYSHCN)*. Office of Emergency Medical Services; 2009. https://oems.nc.gov/wp-content/uploads/2022/10/emschealthcare.pdf. Accessed June 2, 2023.

Northern Virginia EMS Operations Board. *EMS Multiple Casualty Incident Manual*. 2nd ed. Northern Virginia Emergency Response System; 2013.

Office of Health Affairs. *First Responder Guide for Improving Survivability in Improvised Explosive Device and/or Active Shooter Incidents*. U.S. Department of Homeland Security; June 2015. https://www.dhs.gov/sites/default/files/publications/First%20Responder%20Guidance%20June%202015%20FINAL%202_0.pdf. Accessed June 2, 2023.

Schweit KW. *Active Shooter Incidents in the United States in 2014 and 2015*. Federal Bureau of Investigation, U.S. Department of Justice; 2016.

Smith ER Jr, Delaney JB. A new EMS response: supporting paradigm change in EMS operational medical response to active shooter events. *J Emerg Med Serv*. 2013;38(12):48–55. https://www.c-tecc.org/images/content/Smith.Delaney.Active_ShooterDec2013.pdf. Accessed June 2, 2023.

Smith ER Jr, Shapiro G, Sarani B. The profile of wounding in civilian public mass shooting fatalities. *J Trauma Acute Care Surg*. 2016;81(1):86–92.

Texas Engineering Extension Service. *Ambulance Strike Team/Medical Task Force (AST/MTF) Leader. Participant Manual*. Emergency Services Training Institute; 2010.

UPS Foundation. (n.d.). *Managing Spontaneous Volunteers in Times of Disaster: The Synergy of Structure and Good Intentions*. Points of Light Foundation and Volunteer Center National Network. https://www.fema.gov/pdf/donations/ManagingSpontaneousVolunteers.pdf. Accessed June 2, 2023.

U.S. Department of Homeland Security. *Active Shooter: How to Respond*. 2015. https://www.cisa.gov/sites/default/files/publications/active-shooter-how-to-respond-2017-508.pdf. Accessed June 2, 2023.

U.S. Department of Justice, Federal Bureau of Investigation, and the Advanced Law Enforcement Rapid Response Training (ALERRT) Center at Texas State University. *Active Shooter Incidents in the United States in 2022*. U.S. Department of Justice; April 2023.

U.S. Fire Administration. *Emergency Incident Rehabilitation*. Federal Emergency Management Agency; February 2008.

U.S. Fire Administration. *Fire/Emergency Medical Services Department Operational Considerations and Guide for Active Shooter and Mass Casualty Incidents*. Federal Emergency Management Administration; September 2013. https://www.everyonegoeshome.com/wp-content/uploads/2014/04/active_shooter_guide.pdf. Accessed June 2, 2023.

U.S. Fire Administration. *Operational Templates and Guidance for EMS Mass Incident Deployment*. Federal Emergency Management Administration; June 2012. https://www.usfa.fema.gov/downloads/pdf/publications/templates_guidance_ems_mass_incident_deployment.pdf. Accessed June 2, 2023.

Woods GL. *Post Traumatic Stress Symptoms and Critical Stress Debriefing (CISD) in Emergency Medical Services (EMS) Personnel* (Master's Thesis). Available from East Tennessee University, Electronic Theses and Dissertations, Paper 2035. 2007. http://dc.etsu.edu/etd/2035. Accessed June 2, 2023.

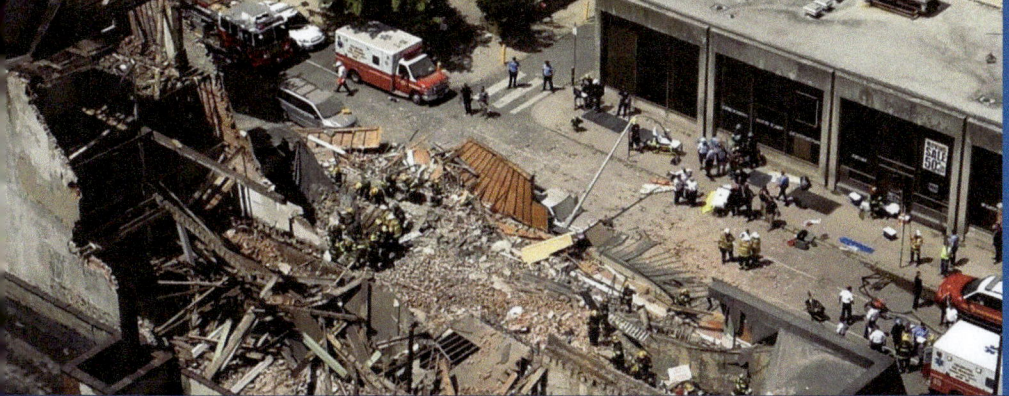

Natural Disasters

LESSON OBJECTIVES

At the completion of this lesson, you should be able to do the following:

· List the different types of natural disasters.

· Identify situations in which shelter in place is preferred over evacuation.

· Discuss management of special needs populations in a natural disaster.

· List the common injuries associated with natural disasters.

· List the potential hazards EMS practitioners can encounter during natural disasters.

Types of Natural Disasters

An environmental phenomenon that will likely negatively impact societies and the human environment is a **natural hazard**. A **natural disaster** refers to the significant harm that befalls a community following a natural hazard. Because most natural hazards can result in a disaster, this course uniformly uses the term *natural disaster*.

The Federal Emergency Management Agency (FEMA) has identified 18 types of natural disasters (**Figure 5-1**). These include hurricanes, tornadoes, tsunamis, earthquakes, coastal and riverine flooding, cold/heat waves, droughts, winter weather, ice storms, landslides, lightning, wildfires, strong winds, and volcanic activity. Most natural disasters are associated with illnesses, injuries, loss of life, damaged infrastructure (e.g., power outages, transportation disruptions), and food and water supply shortages. Sometimes one natural disaster acts as a precursor to another natural disaster. For example, earthquakes can cause tsunamis, and drought, heat waves, and lightning are often associated with wildfires. It is also possible for a natural disaster to cause a

technologic disaster, as in 2011 when a nuclear reactor in Japan experienced a meltdown following a tsunami, which was triggered by an earthquake.

The Impact of Natural Disasters

According to the World Meteorological Association, between 1970 and 2019, weather, climate, and water hazards accounted for 50% of all disasters, 45% of all reported disaster-related deaths, and 74% of all reported economic losses.

Warned Natural Disaster

In the United States, 90% of natural disasters involve flooding. Certain natural hazards, such as hurricanes, winter weather, heat waves, droughts, and flooding, can be detected prior to occurring and we can be "warned"; hence the term **warned natural disasters**. A **warning** means that a severe weather event has been detected

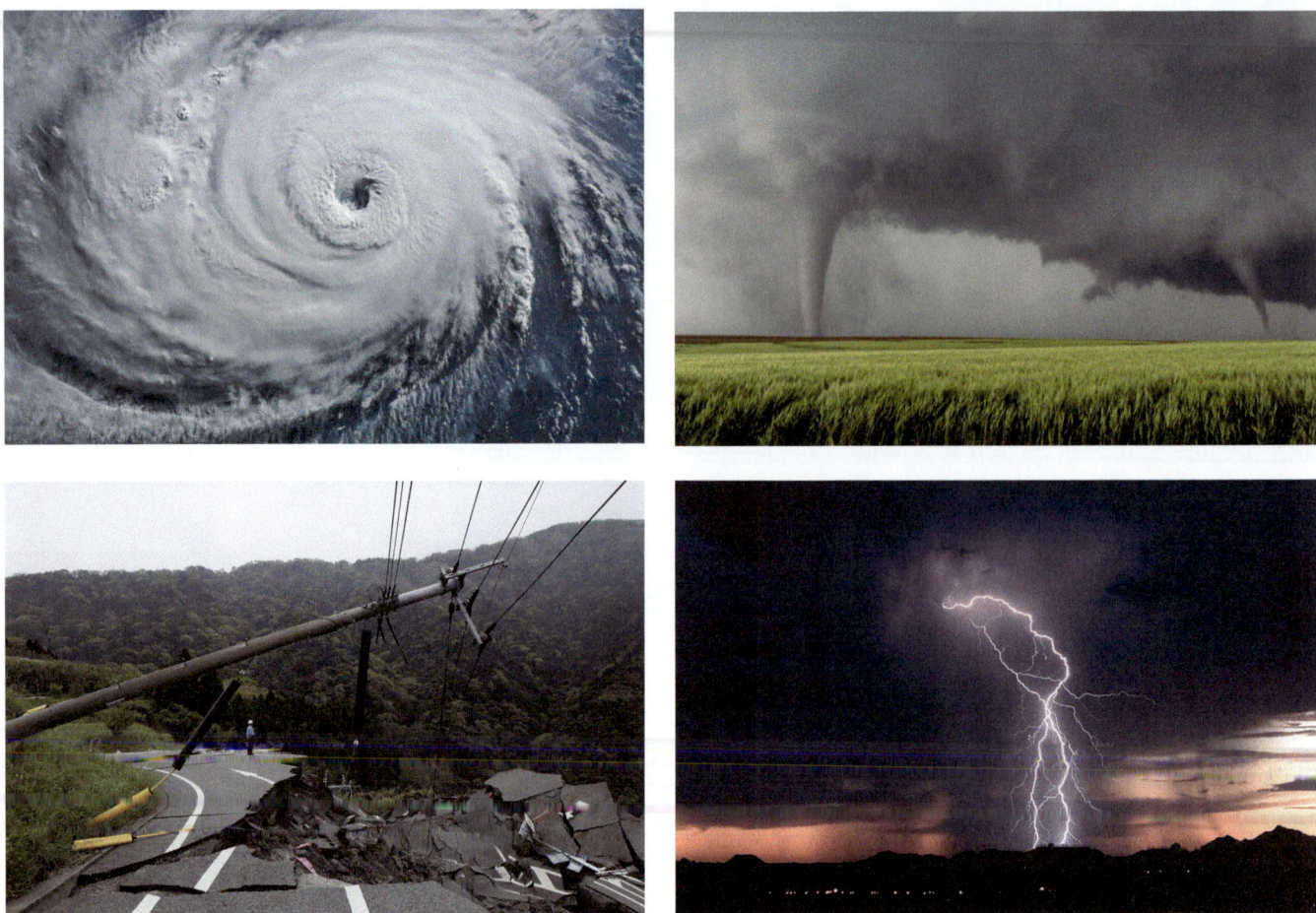

Figure 5-1 FEMA has identified 18 types of natural disasters, including hurricanes, tornadoes, lightning strikes, and landslides.

© flashpict/Shutterstock; © Huntstyle/Shutterstock; © austinding/Shutterstock; © Jhaz Photography/Shutterstock

and is approaching (e.g., funnel clouds have formed or a tornado has touched down). The amount of warning time varies based on the type of natural hazard. For example, there may only be a few minutes of lead time before a tornado, whereas there are often several days of awareness before a hurricane. Advance warning of a natural hazard allows time for officials and the community to mitigate the effects of the natural hazard by taking such steps as educating the public, evacuation planning, boarding windows/doors, stocking supplies, restricting travel, and conserving resources.

A concept closely related to a warning is a watch. A severe weather **watch** means conditions exist and are favorable for a severe weather event, though no active threat to the community has been detected. Public education about severe weather forecasting (i.e., watches versus warnings) has been particularly effective at saving lives; however, the public has sometimes had difficulty understanding the difference between a watch and a warning. In 2021, the Normal, Illinois, fire department posted an image to their Facebook page to help

community members understand the difference between a watch and a warning, using tacos as a metaphor for severe weather (**Figure 5-2**). This campaign has since gone viral and is a great example of how EMS can help communicate complex concepts to the public.

No-Notice Natural Disasters

Some natural disasters, such as earthquakes, volcanic activity, wildfires, avalanches, tsunamis, and landslides, often occur with little to no warning; these are called **no-notice natural disasters**. Due to their unexpected nature, only preparedness actions that the community has taken for months/years before the disaster can mitigate their effects. These preparedness actions include enacting strict building codes and zoning based on the topography, planting trees to strengthen soil and make it less prone to erosion, and ensuring sustainable development (i.e., balancing the natural landscape with the construction/infrastructure needs of a growing population).

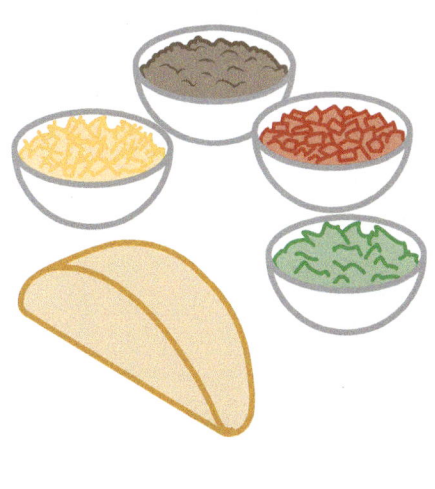

Taco Watch

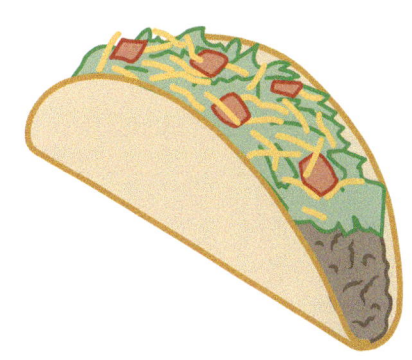

Taco Warning

Figure 5-2 Watch versus warning.
© National Association of Emergency Medical Technicians (NAEMT)

Evacuation in a Natural Disaster

Evacuation is the timely and rapid movement of people exposed to actual/imminent danger in a disaster to safer locations and places of shelter in order to protect them. Evacuation is commonly characterized by a short time frame, from hours to weeks, within which emergency procedures must be enacted to save lives and minimize exposure to harm. Hundreds to millions of people may need to evacuate quickly in case of natural disasters such as hurricanes, floods, earthquakes, and wildfires.

It is important to note that evacuation may be done before a disaster (such as before a hurricane makes landfall) or following a disaster to help redistribute patients (**Figure 5-3**). Evacuation can refer to a nonpatient population (e.g., a community in a geographic area) or a patient/cohort (e.g., ICU patients).

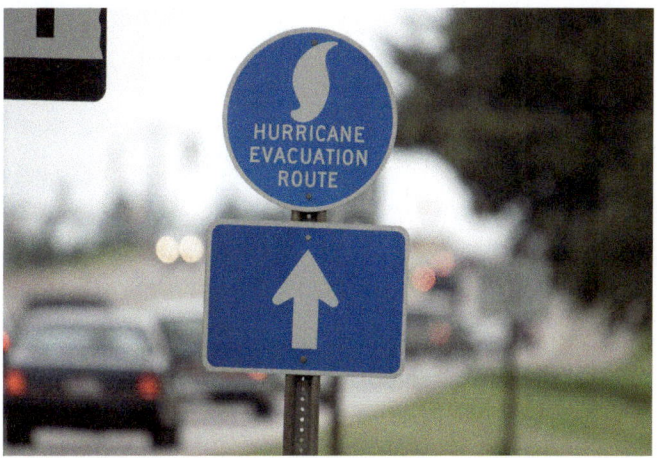

Figure 5-3 A road sign intended to guide evacuees to a safe location.
© Tad Denson/Shutterstock

Psychological and Social Impact of Evacuation

People displaced from their homes by disasters, including evacuees, often face health risks due to the altered living conditions (e.g., separation from social support and familiar resources for meeting basic needs). Research shows that long-term psychological and social harm affects individuals after evacuation, particularly when they cannot return to their original homes. Evacuees can suffer up to twice the illness rate compared to others affected by an emergency but not dislocated from their homes and communities. In some areas, this impact is further exacerbated by the constant threat of evacuation due to the increasing severity and frequency of natural disasters.

Phases of Evacuation

The phases of an evacuation include an evacuation warning and an immediate evacuation order (**Figure 5-4**). **Evacuation warning** is the official term for the alert issued to people in an area that faces a potential threat to life and property. It considers the probability that an area will be affected and prepares people for a potential immediate evacuation order. This warning is often associated

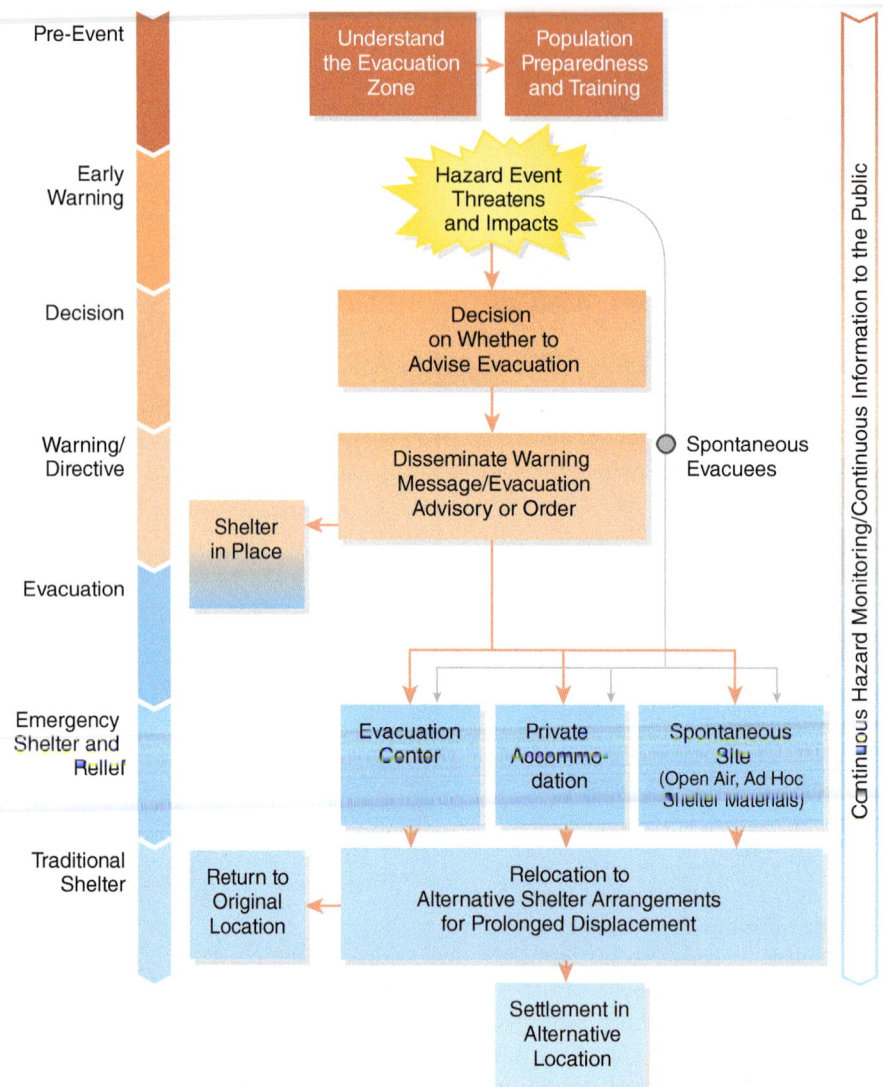

Figure 5-4 Evacuation phases.

Data from Internal Displacement Monitoring Centre. Global Estimates 2012: People Displaced by Disasters. Internal Displacement Monitoring Centre; 2013.

with the term *voluntary evacuation* by the media. People who need additional time should consider evacuating when the warning is issued rather than waiting for an immediate evacuation order.

An **immediate evacuation order** requires the immediate movement of people out of an affected area due to an imminent threat to life (**Figure 5-5**). Choosing to stay could result in loss of life and impede emergency personnel's work. In a rapidly developing emergency, an immediate evacuation order may be the only warning people in the affected area receive. This order is often associated with the term *mandatory evacuation* by the media. The evacuation announcement should involve activation of the Emergency Alert System, use of traditional and social media, and door-to-door messaging.

Sheltering in Place vs. Evacuation

In some situations, **sheltering in place** may be the preferred option to avoid exposure to outside environmental hazards, such as radiologic or airborne contaminants, storm surges, and high wind. The decision to shelter in place requires an organized method of securing building entrances, including windows and ventilation systems, to prevent outside environmental hazards from entering the building. Building and safety personnel, homeowners, and residents should have contingencies to move to and/or create safe rooms and designated safe areas if sheltering in place is recommended. FEMA provides the public with sheltering-in-place guidance for 10 hazards and three building types (mobile homes, one- or two-story

Richard Cordova
Fire Captain
CAL FIRE *Southern Region*
Public Education/Public Information Officer
Cell: 951-337-3673
RCordova@fire.ca.gov

CAL FIRE NEWS RELEASE
California Department of Forestry and Fire Protection

CONTACT:	Information Line: (831) 204-0446	**RELEASE DATE:**	July 24, 2016
		TIME: 9:00 p.m.	

Mandatory Evacuation Orders Expand on Soberanes Fire

The Monterey County Sheriff's Department has expanded the mandatory evacuation order to include:

- *Rocky Creek*
- *Weston Ridge Road (AKA Garrapata Ridge Road)*
- *Palo Colorado Road*
- *Highway 1 @ Old Coast Road south to Old Coast Road @ Bixby Creek Road*
- *Garrapatos Road*

    All residents are required to evacuate the designated area immediately!

Evacuation advisories remain in place for:

- Community of Carmel Highlands
- South of Rancho San Carlos
- White Rock
- Old Coast Road south from Bixby Creek Road to Little Sur River

Residents are asked to be READY: Create and maintain defensible space and harden your home against flying embers. Get SET: Prepare your family and home ahead of time for the possibility of having to evacuate. Be Ready to GO! Take the evacuation steps necessary to give your family and home the best chance of surviving a wildfire.

For more information on Ready, Set, Go, go to www.readyforwildfire.org .

Residents should be prepared to leave the area immediately if a Voluntary or Mandatory Evacuation Order is issued. If you evacuate be sure to take any medications, pets, family valuables etc. with you, close all windows including window coverings, and leave all doors closed. A temporary shelter facility has been established at the Carmel Middle School 4380 Carmel Valley Road. For further information dial 2-1-1.

For additional information on the Soberanes Fire, Monterey County residents should contact Soberanes Fire Information Line at (831) 204-0446. Or visit CAL FIRE online @ www.fire.ca.gov .

###

Figure 5-5 Evacuation order issued by the Santa Barbara County Sherriff's Department in California.

Courtesy of the California Department of Forestry and Fire Protection

buildings, and multistory buildings; **Figure 5-6**). This guidance includes recommended interior locations by hazard, additional protective actions, and duration.

Vulnerable Patients/ Special Needs Population

The National Response Framework (NRF) defines members of a special needs population as individuals with needs before, during, and after an incident in the following functional areas: maintaining independence, communication, transportation, supervision, and medical care. In addition to people with needs in these functional areas, the special needs population includes individuals with service animals or pets. As of 2023, 66% of all U.S. households have pets. Notably, thousands of the people who did not evacuate during Hurricane Katrina chose to remain with their animals.

Maintaining Independence

Individuals who rely on assistance to maintain their independence in daily activities may lose this support during a disaster. This disruption may affect their ability to obtain supplies (e.g., diapers, formula, catheters, ostomy supplies), effectively use durable medical equipment (e.g., wheelchairs, walkers), and/or receive assistance from attendants or caregivers.

Communication

Some individuals have hearing, vision, speech, cognitive, or intellectual limitations and/or limited English proficiency that prevents them from hearing verbal announcements, seeing directional signs, or understanding how to obtain assistance. Community resources must be prepared to effectively disseminate emergency information to this population.

Transportation

Some individuals are unable to drive or do not have a vehicle. During an evacuation, they may require transportation support, including accessible vehicles (e.g., lift-equipped vehicles, vehicles suitable for transporting individuals who use oxygen) or help accessing mass transportation (**Figure 5-7**).

Caregivers and Chaperons

Some individuals, such as those with dementia or a psychiatric condition, require assistance to adapt to a new environment. Young children who are separated from their caregivers may not have the cognitive ability to recognize and respond appropriately to dangers. Community emergency services should identify people who would need help during an evacuation and coordinate with appropriate resources to form an action plan.

Medical Care

Individuals who have unstable, terminal, or contagious conditions may rely on medical assistance, including ongoing treatment and monitoring. Their needs may include intravenous therapy, tube feeding, dialysis, oxygen administration, airway maintenance, wound management, and the operation of life-sustaining equipment that may present power and technology challenges during a disaster. Again, communities must identify these individuals in advance and coordinate with appropriate resources to form an action plan.

Identifying Vulnerable Patients

The Department of Health and Human Services (HHS) provides a planning resource to identify vulnerable populations in each community. The HHS emPOWER Map identifies Medicare beneficiaries who live independently but rely on electricity-dependent equipment and other

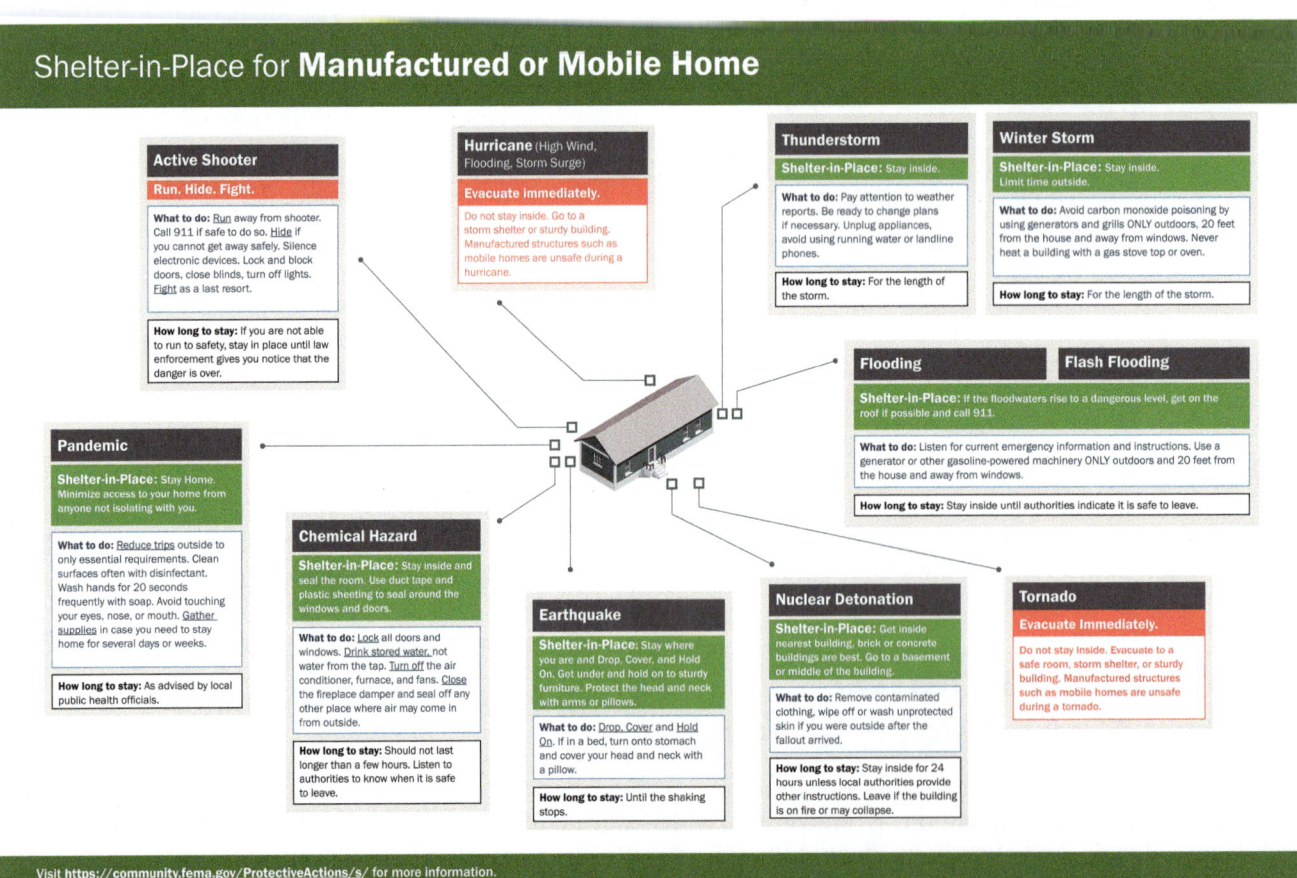

A.

Figure 5-6 **A.** FEMA shelter-in-place guidance for individuals in a manufactured or mobile home during hurricane conditions.

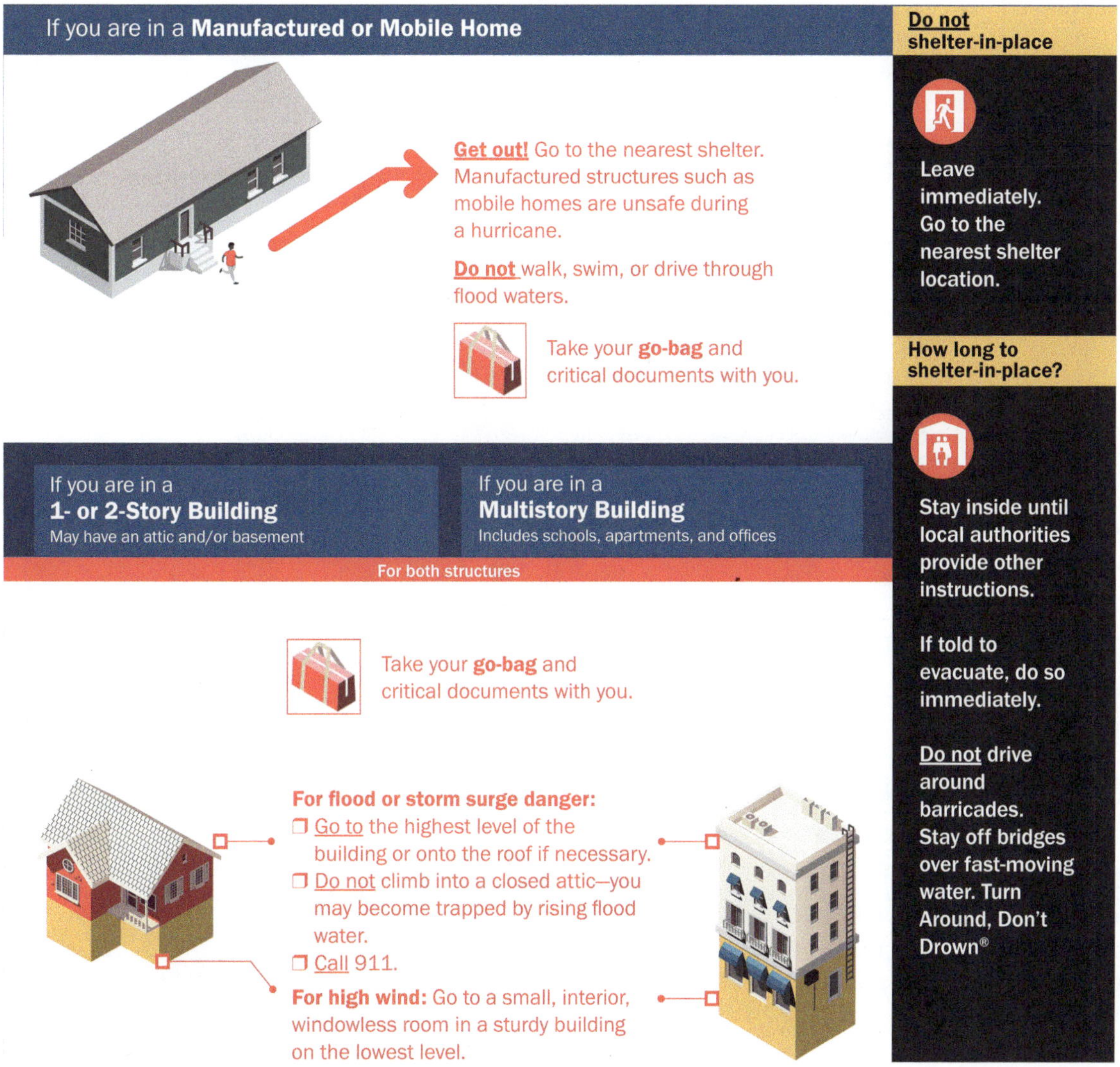

If you are in a **Manufactured or Mobile Home**

Get out! Go to the nearest shelter. Manufactured structures such as mobile homes are unsafe during a hurricane.

Do not walk, swim, or drive through flood waters.

Take your **go-bag** and critical documents with you.

Do not shelter-in-place

Leave immediately. Go to the nearest shelter location.

How long to shelter-in-place?

Stay inside until local authorities provide other instructions.

If told to evacuate, do so immediately.

Do not drive around barricades. Stay off bridges over fast-moving water. Turn Around, Don't Drown®

If you are in a **1- or 2-Story Building**
May have an attic and/or basement

If you are in a **Multistory Building**
Includes schools, apartments, and offices

For both structures

Take your **go-bag** and critical documents with you.

For flood or storm surge danger:
☐ Go to the highest level of the building or onto the roof if necessary.
☐ Do not climb into a closed attic—you may become trapped by rising flood water.
☐ Call 911.

For high wind: Go to a small, interior, windowless room in a sturdy building on the lowest level.

B.

Figure 5-6 B. FEMA shelter-in-place guidance for those in a multistory building during different disaster types. *(continued)*

Reproduced from Federal Emergency Management Agency. FEMA shelter-in-place pictogram. Published November 2021. https://www.fema.gov/sites/default/files/documents/fema_shelter-in-place_guidance.pdf

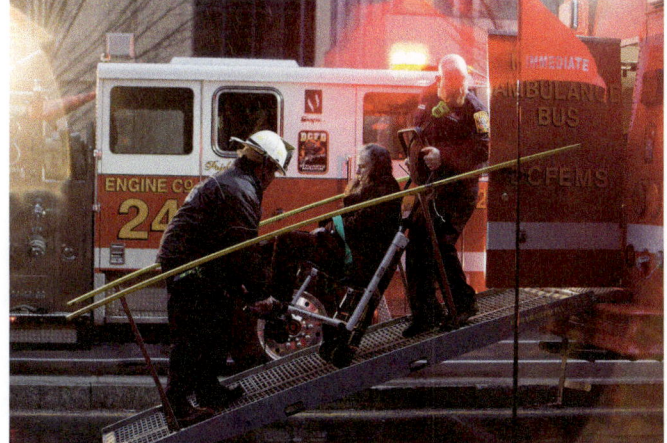

Figure 5-7 Some individuals will require special transportation services during evacuation.
© Jacquelyn Martin/AP Photo

health care resources. These individuals are at particular risk during a disaster. Responders can use this resource to help ensure emergency preparedness, response, and recovery (**Figure 5-8**). It is available at the Public Health Emergency HHS emPOWER Map website (https://empowerprogram.hhs.gov/empowermap).

Destination Determination

During a larger disaster in the community, it is best not to overload the hospital with nonacute patients. Alternative dispositions should be considered based on community emergency response plans and applicable regulations. Depending on community emergency response plans and applicable regulations, evacuees might be transported by ambulance to a shelter or a special medical needs shelter. **Special medical needs shelters** are designed to keep displaced noninstitutionalized individuals

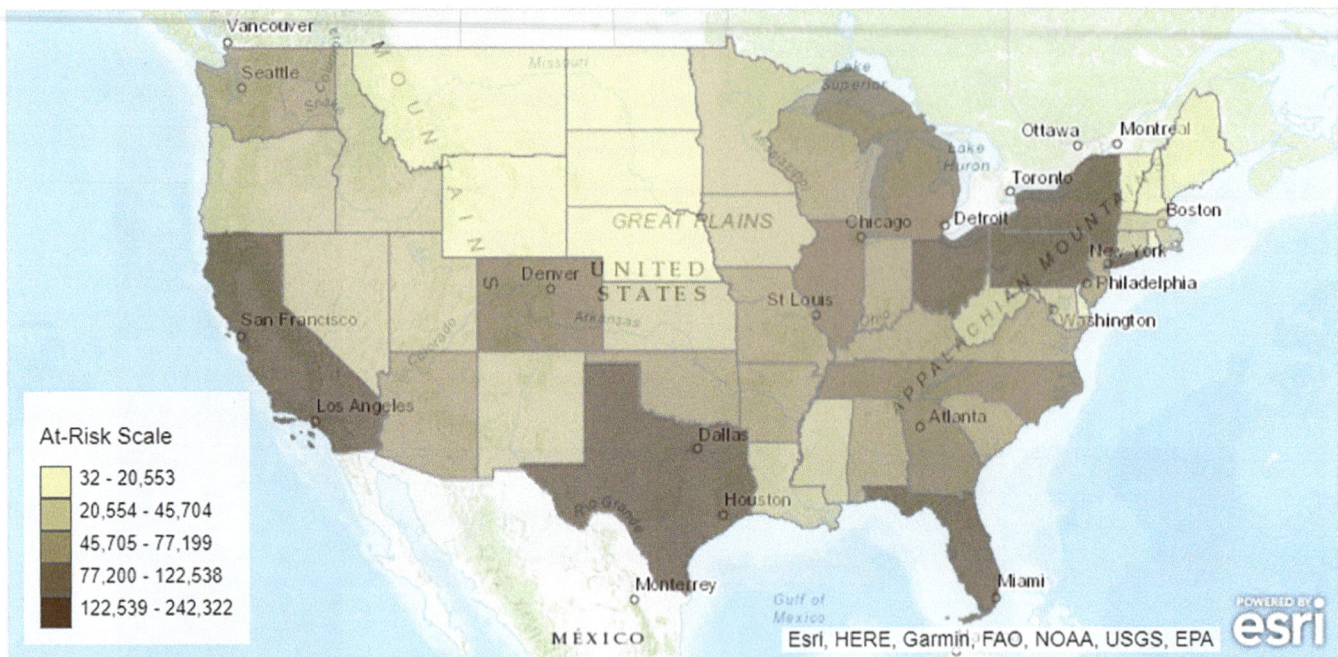

Figure 5-8 HHS emPOWER Map.
Courtesy of the U.S. Department of Health and Human Services

Essential Items to be Brought with the Special Needs Patient During Evacuation/Relocation

Emergency responders must bring the following essential items with special needs patients during evacuation/relocation:

- Medications
- Oxygen supply
- Nasal cannula and tubing
- Home nebulizer and continuous positive airway pressure (CPAP) machines
- Walkers, wheelchairs, and other ambulatory aids
- Hearing aids (and chargers)
- Glasses
- Medical records
- Service animal (and supplies)
- Nonservice animals (based on local practice)

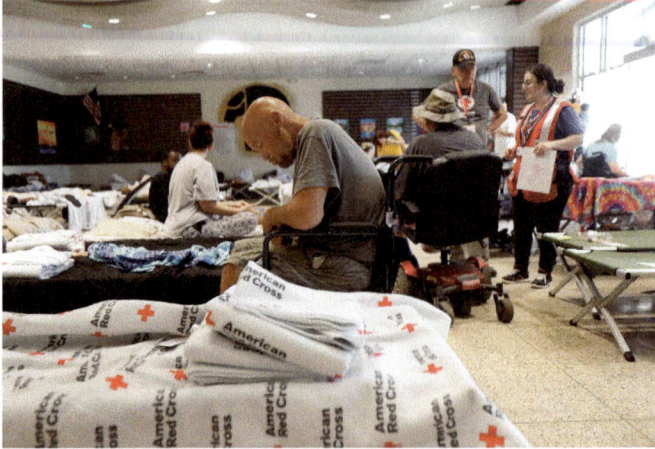

Figure 5-9 Individuals who need assistance with activities of daily living may benefit from a special medical needs shelter when displaced from their homes during a disaster.
© Gerald Herbert/AP Photo

who need assistance with activities of daily living out of a hospital setting during an emergency (**Figure 5-9**). They may aid with oxygen administration, blood glucose monitoring, basic wound care, and medication compliance. Higher-acuity patients may be cared for in the out-of-hospital environment based on the capabilities of the local jurisdiction or resources brought in for the response (such as a disaster medical assistance team).

Potential Hazards for EMS and Local Populations

Emergency responders face many potential hazards during natural disasters. Traditional transport routes could be rendered unusable due to debris, collapsed roadways, flooding, and downed trees or electric wires/poles. Downed electric wires and poles could pose additional challenges if they remain energized. Electricity outages would impact the care and services EMS can

Common Injuries/Illnesses in Specific Natural Disasters

Specific natural disasters are associated with certain common injuries and illnesses.

Hurricanes/Floods

- Infection from water that has been contaminated by sewage or toxic chemicals
- Infected wounds caused by airborne or floating debris
- Injuries from fallen trees, motor vehicle collisions, or debris impact
- Mosquito-borne infections from standing water
- Hypothermia

Tornadoes

- Head trauma
- Soft-tissue injuries
- Fractures

Wildfires

- Irritation to the eyes, airway, and respiratory system
- Injuries from debris, including head injuries and lacerations
- Burns
- Esophageal inhalation injuries
- Electrical hazards
- Rashes

- Infections
- Exposure to toxic substances

Earthquakes

- Injuries due to falling objects or building collapse
- Lacerations
- Fractures
- Head trauma
- Abdominal injuries
- Crush syndrome

Severe Winter Weather

- Frostbite/frostnip
- Hypothermia

Excessive Heat Events

- Heat edema
- Heat cramps
- Heat exhaustion
- Heatstroke
- Dehydration

Lightning Strikes

- Cardiac arrest
- Traumatic injuries
- Neurologic defects

provide during natural disasters. Natural disasters could impact medical care facilities, creating the additional problem of determining where to transport patients needing definitive medical care. Atmospheric contamination by itself could pose health hazards to responding EMS practitioners.

Local populations face additional challenges during natural disasters (**Figure 5-10**). These include injuries, animal- and insect-related hazards (e.g., mosquito bites), safe cleanup, food and drinking water safety, carbon monoxide poisoning, illness from sewage, temperature-related illnesses, infectious disease outbreaks, wound-related problems, and mental health issues.

Common Injuries

Natural disasters are commonly associated with injuries and illnesses, including blunt trauma, orthopedic injuries, crush injuries/crush syndrome, and exacerbation of existing medical conditions.

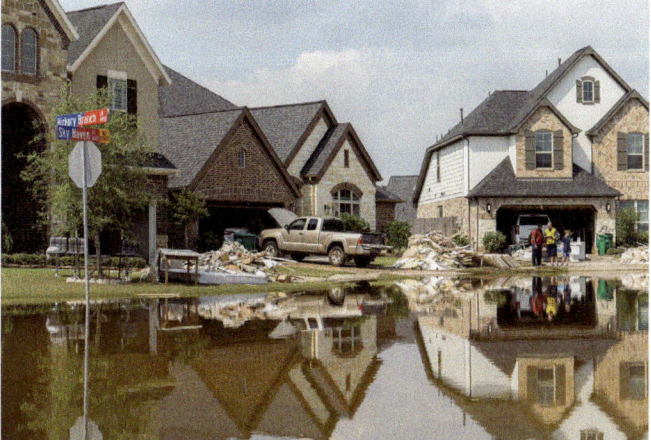

Figure 5-10 Local populations may face various challenges during a natural disaster.
© michelmond/Shutterstock

Blunt Trauma

Blunt trauma results from compression or **shear forces.** In a natural disaster, falling objects/structural collapses, mechanical falls, and crashing into objects could result in blunt trauma. Recognition of major internal injuries, immediate stabilization of life-threatening injuries, rapid transport, and prompt en-route care are critical to survival.

Orthopedic Injuries

In a natural disaster, orthopedic injuries are common (**Figure 5-11**). Management of open fractures involves rinsing open wounds or exposed bone ends with saline or sterile water, covering them with a moistened sterile dressing, and considering pain medication. To manage amputations, the focus must be on hemorrhage control.

Crush Injuries/Crush Syndrome

Crushed extremity injuries are common in natural disasters such as earthquakes, hurricanes, and tornadoes. Crush injuries can cause rhabdomyolysis due to the

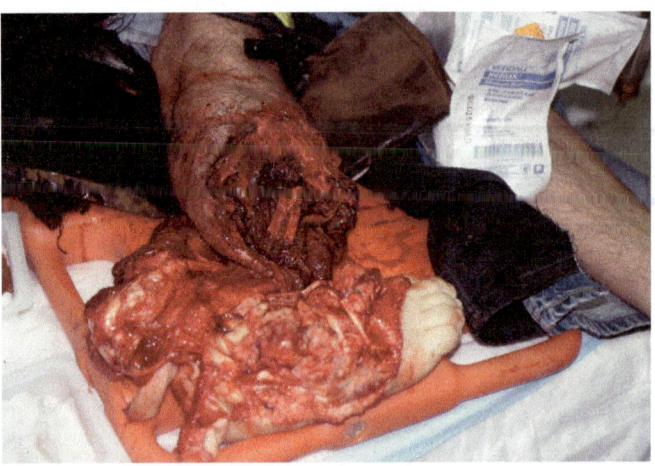

A.

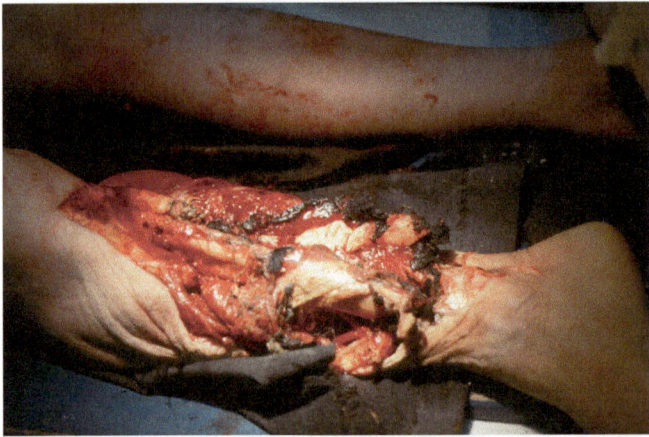

B.

Figure 5-11 A. Complete amputation of the right leg after it became entangled in machinery. **B.** Mangled extremity resulting from crushing injury between two vehicles. The patient has fractures and extensive soft-tissue injury.

Courtesy of Peter T. Pons, MD, FACEP

associated muscle death and release of myoglobin. Rhabdomyolysis is prevalent in patients who have experienced prolonged entrapment, traumatic injury to muscle mass, and compromised circulation to the injured area. Early and aggressive fluid resuscitation is critical to improve patient outcomes. Advanced life support (ALS) personnel need to monitor closely for signs of hyperkalemia and be prepared to provide treatment. Patient resuscitation, including fluid administration, should begin prior to extrication; otherwise, the patient may go into cardiac arrest during extrication following the sudden release of metabolic by-products and potassium into the bloodstream when the compression of the extremity is released.

Exacerbation of Medical Conditions

Disruption in the power supply during a natural disaster can lead to a gap in medical services or care that relies on electricity. This disruption can affect medical procedures, refrigeration of medications such as insulin, and medical devices such as CPAP machines. Natural disasters are also associated with exacerbation of chronic medical conditions. Chronic physical health conditions such as diabetes, heart failure, hypertension, chronic obstructive pulmonary disease (COPD), acute bronchitis, and asthma are worsened, especially for patients without access to prescription medications. Chronic mental health conditions that may be exacerbated by natural disasters include depression, alcohol and substance overuse, interpersonal violence, posttraumatic stress disorder (PTSD) or anxiety disorders, and schizophrenia.

Triage and Transport in Natural Disasters

Triage concepts for injuries are unchanged in natural disasters, in that patients with life-threatening injuries are given the highest treatment priority. As the disaster progresses, there are often more medical patients who must also be managed and triaged. Larger and prolonged disasters can also contain mass-casualty events within them. For example, during evacuation from a hurricane, a bus of evacuees overturns, leading to a mass-casualty incident (MCI).

A natural disaster could be associated with transport challenges, including long transport times. These could be due to infrastructure conditions (damaged roads), downed power lines, uprooted trees blocking roadways, collapsed buildings, and flooding. Patients may need to be transported by various means, such as ambulances, helicopters, planes, boats, customized buses, and mass transit vehicles (for ambulatory patients). Air medical can be an option if in a remote area; in urban areas, ground transport may be better.

Patient Tracking

Patients should be tracked through an emergency operations center, a multiple-agency coordination center, or a health care evacuation center. EMS practitioners can use methods to preserve essential medical information with each evacuee, including transporting printed medical records with the patient or using electronic medical records via a regional health information organization. The National Disaster Medical System (NDMS) Joint Patient Assessment Tracking System (JPATS) tracks all federal patient movement during a disaster. This includes patients who are moved/evacuated, are admitted to a federally supported shelter, or are receiving NDMS-definitive care at local facilities. Local and regional EMS systems should consider how patient-tracking mechanisms could be ensured in the setting of communications/technology/infrastructure loss.

Public Education

Communitywide awareness and education programs about natural disasters are critical in reducing loss of life, personal injuries, and property damage from natural disasters. Such programs must consider all sections of the population, including small children, older adults, people with disabilities, and those with limited English proficiency. Programs should address educational needs at the following levels:

- *Household*: Provide information on household survival plans, precautionary measures, emergency supplies, and prescription medications.
- *Community*: Promote planning, education, and preparedness actions by hospitals, civic organizations, faith-based groups, schools, businesses, neighborhood organizations, and community groups.
- *Schools*: Teach information on natural disaster preparedness, warnings, and response.
- *Institutions of higher learning*: Incorporate disaster impact education for all relevant professions.
- *Workplace*: Ensure the safety and security of workers and business assets.
- *Public officials and news media*: Ensure that procedures are in place to inform the public before, during, and after a disaster.
- *First responders*: Provide continuing education, exercises, and simulations related to disaster response.

Preparedness

Preparedness or mitigation programs can help reduce the impact of natural disasters through the following efforts:

- Constructing and locating schools, government buildings, and hospitals to avoid or withstand natural hazards

- Strengthening existing medical and educational facilities
- Adopting nonstructural measures (such as not storing perishable supplies on the ground level)
- Incorporating mitigation into new facility design development
- Protecting cultural properties and natural resources
- Involving government leadership at all levels in the design, location, and construction of hazard-resistant facilities
- Providing training programs
- Conducting research on strategies for and barriers to the implementation of mitigation strategies for all natural hazards

Personal Preparedness

Just as each community and agency must undertake a comprehensive planning process to be prepared for the challenges of a potential disaster, each prehospital care practitioner must be ready to face, on a personal and professional level, the many issues the disaster may present.

Prehospital care practitioners must understand the many potential hazards that may accompany a disaster response before the actual incident and be prepared to take the necessary steps to protect themselves from these dangers. Gaps in knowledge about such issues as building collapse, hazardous materials incidents, active shooter/hostile events, weapons of mass destruction (WMDs) and their potential effects on patient treatment, appropriate personal protective equipment (PPE), and overall incident management should be addressed in advance. Regular training and interagency drills are proactive ways to maintain skills and competencies and practice a concerted response with first responders of different disciplines.

Disasters may extend beyond a typical operating period, and prehospital care practitioners must discuss their roles, responsibilities, and potentially prolonged absence with their families. This discussion includes preparing their families for what they should do and where they should go during such an event to ensure their safety. Just as the local EMS system procures supplies and equipment before a disaster, practitioners should ensure that adequate supplies are available at home to meet their families' needs. Practitioners should plan for who would care for children and pets during an extended tour of duty. Taking these actions will help reassure both the practitioner and family members, allowing the practitioner to continue operating during a disaster if needed, especially during an extended response.

An additional resource with information about personal and family preparation in the event of a disaster, including how to create a family communication plan, is the Ready campaign sponsored by FEMA, available online at www.ready.gov.

Emergency Supply List

All homes should have some basic supplies on hand (at least 3 days' worth) for emergencies. The following is a list of some basic items that emergency supply kits should include. It is important that individuals review this list and consider where they live and the unique needs of their family to create an emergency supply kit that will meet their specific needs. Individuals should also consider having at least two emergency supply kits, one full kit at home and smaller portable kits in their workplace, vehicle, or other places where they spend time. Prescription medications are also an important consideration when planning one's emergency kit.

- Water—1 gallon per person and pet, per day (3-day supply for evacuation, 2-week supply for home)
  - Consider storing more water than this for hot climates, for pregnant women, and for persons who are sick.
  - Consider adding an effective water filter.
- Food—nonperishable, easy-to-prepare items, including food for pets (3-day supply for evacuation, 2-week supply for home)
  - Remember, it is better to have extra food that you can share than to run out of food during an emergency.
- Cell phone with chargers and rechargeable battery packs
- Battery-powered or hand-cranked radio and a National Oceanic and Atmospheric Administration (NOAA) weather radio with tone alert and extra batteries for both
- Flashlight and extra batteries
- First aid kit
- Whistle to signal for help
- Dust mask to help filter contaminated air and plastic sheeting and duct tape to shelter in place
- Moist towelettes, garbage bags, and plastic ties for personal sanitation
- Wrench or pliers to turn off utilities (or multitool device that includes both)
- Can opener for food (if kit contains nonperishable food)
- Local maps

Additional items to consider adding to an emergency supply kit:

- *Items for infants*, including formula, diapers, bottles, pacifiers, powdered milk, and medications not requiring refrigeration
- *Items for seniors, persons with special needs, or anyone with serious allergies*, including special foods, denture items, extra eyeglasses, hearing aid batteries, prescription and nonprescription medications that are regularly used, inhalers, and other essential equipment
- Prescription medications and glasses
- Important family documents such as copies of insurance policies, identification, important medical records, and bank account records in a waterproof, portable container
- Cash and change
- Emergency reference material such as a first aid book or information from FEMA's Ready campaign (www.ready.gov)
- Sleeping bag or warm blanket for each person (Consider additional bedding if you live in a cold-weather climate.)
- Complete change of clothing, including a long-sleeved shirt, long pants, and sturdy shoes (Consider additional clothing if you live in a cold-weather climate.)
- Household chlorine bleach and medicine dropper (A diluted solution of 9 parts water to 1 part bleach can be used as a disinfectant. In an emergency, bleach can be used to treat water by mixing 16 drops of regular household liquid bleach per gallon of water; do not use bleaches that are scented or color safe or that have added cleaners.)
- Fire extinguisher (A-B-C type)
- Matches in a waterproof container

- Paper and pencil
- Entertainment—including games and books, favorite toys, and stuffed animals for small children
- Kitchen accessories—a manual can opener; mess kits or disposable cups, plates, and utensils; utility knife; salt and sugar; aluminum foil and plastic wrap; resealable plastic bags; paper towels
- Sanitation and hygiene items—shampoo, deodorant, toothpaste, toothbrushes, comb and brush, lip balm, sunscreen, contact lenses and supplies, any medications regularly used, toilet paper, moist towelettes, soap, hand sanitizer, liquid detergent, feminine supplies, plastic garbage bags (heavy duty) and ties (for personal sanitation uses), medium-sized plastic bucket with tight lid, disinfectant, household chlorine bleach
- Needles and thread
- A map of the area marked with places you could go and their telephone numbers (including phone numbers for out-of-town family members)
- An extra set of keys and IDs—including keys for cars and any properties owned and copies of driver's licenses, passports, and work identification badges
- Copies of credit cards
- Copies of medical prescriptions
- A small tent, compass, and shovel

Pack the items in easy-to-carry containers, such as a 5-gallon bucket, label the containers clearly, and store them where they would be easily accessible. Duffle bags, backpacks, and covered trash receptacles are good candidates for containers. In a disaster situation, a family may need access to the disaster supply kit quickly—whether sheltering at home or evacuating. Ensuring that family vehicles are filled with gasoline and electric vehicles are charged will allow for immediate evacuation to a safe location. Following a disaster, having the right supplies can help a household endure sheltering in place or evacuation.

Make sure the needs of everyone who would use the kit are covered, including infants, seniors, and pets. It is a good idea to involve whoever may use the kit, including children, in assembling it. Kits should be updated yearly to account for children's growth and development as well as changes to prescriptions and review of expiration dates.

Source: Modified from Federal Emergency Management Agency. Ready America. n.d. www.ready.gov, https://www.ready.gov/kit; and Centers for Disease Control and Prevention. All-Hazards Preparedness Guide. n.d. https://www.cdc.gov/cpr /documents/AHPG_FINAL_March_2013.pdf

Food Kit

- Store at least a 3-day supply of nonperishable food.
- Select foods that require no refrigeration, preparation, or cooking and little or no water.
- Pack a manual can opener and eating utensils.
- Avoid salty foods, as they will make you thirsty.
- Choose foods your family will eat.
- Suggested foods include the following:
  - Ready-to-eat canned meats, fruits, and vegetables
  - Protein or fruit bars
  - Dry cereal or granola
  - Peanut butter
  - Dried fruit
  - Nuts
  - Crackers
  - Canned juices
  - Nonperishable pasteurized milk
  - High-energy foods
  - Vitamins
  - Food for infants
  - Comfort/stress foods
- Bring a propane stove or grill for cooking (with extra propane tank).

Source: Data from Federal Emergency Management Agency. Ready America. n.d. www.ready.gov; and Centers for Disease Control and Prevention. Emergency Preparedness and Response. n.d. https://emergency.cdc.gov/

First Aid Kit

In any emergency, a family member may be cut or burned or may suffer other injuries. An emergency kit should include the following:

- Two pairs of latex gloves or other sterile gloves (if anyone has latex allergies)
- Sterile dressings and a commercial (as opposed to an improvised) tourniquet to stop bleeding
- Cleansing agent/soap and antibiotic towelettes to disinfect
- Antibiotic ointment to prevent infection
- Burn ointment to prevent infection
- Adhesive bandages in a variety of sizes
- Eye wash solution to flush the eyes or to use as a general decontaminant
- Thermometer
- Daily prescription medications such as insulin, cardiac medications, and asthma inhalers (Periodically rotate medicines to account for expiration dates.)
- Prescribed medical supplies such as glucose and blood pressure monitoring equipment and supplies
- Any durable medical equipment like canes or walkers (special thought should be given to powering durable medical equipment [e.g., ventilator, CPAP machine, scooter, chair lift] during a power outage)

Other useful items to include:
- Cell phone with charger
- Scissors
- Tweezers
- Tube of petroleum jelly or other lubricant
- Nonprescription medications:
  - Aspirin or nonaspirin pain reliever (acetaminophen)
  - Antidiarrheal medication
  - Antacid (for upset stomach)
  - Laxative

Source: Data from Federal Emergency Management Agency. Ready America. n.d. www.ready.gov; and Centers for Disease Control and Prevention. Emergency Preparedness and Response. n.d. https://emergency.cdc.gov/

SUMMARY

- A natural disaster results from significant harm to a community following a natural hazard.
- Preparedness actions that the community has taken in prior months or years can mitigate the effects of no-notice or unexpected natural disasters.
- Warnings provided in advance of certain natural disasters can allow individuals and the community to take steps to mitigate the disaster's effects. Such steps include evacuating, shuttering, stocking supplies, restricting travel, and conserving resources.
- Evacuation in natural disasters refers to the timely and rapid movement of people exposed to actual/imminent danger to safer locations and places of shelter.
- Sheltering in place is preferable to evacuation in certain natural disasters to avoid exposure to outside environmental hazards, radiologic/airborne contaminants, storm surges, and high wind.
- The vulnerable population includes individuals with service animals or pets and those with needs before, during, and after an incident in the following functional areas: maintaining independence, communication, transportation, supervision, and medical care.
- EMS practitioners must avoid overloading hospitals with nonacute patients!
- Special medical needs shelters can often assist with oxygen, blood glucose monitoring, basic wound care, and medication compliance.
- EMS practitioners face potential hazards during natural disasters: traditional EMS transport routes rendered unusable, downed electric wires/poles, electricity outages, debris, medical care facilities impacted, and atmospheric contamination.
- Common injuries associated with natural disasters include blunt trauma, orthopedic injuries, crush injuries/crush syndrome, and exacerbation of medical conditions.
- Triage concepts for injuries are unchanged in natural disasters.
- Patients should be tracked through an emergency operations center, a multiple-agency coordination center, or a health care evacuation center.
- Natural disasters take a psychological toll on both the victims and EMS practitioners.
- Communitywide awareness and education programs about natural disasters are critical in reducing loss of life, personal injuries, and property damage from natural disasters.

References and Additional Resources

Abt Associates Inc. *Estimating Loss of Life From Hurricane-Related Flooding in the Greater New Orleans Area: Health Effects of Hurricane Katrina.* Abt Associates; May 2006.

Agency for Healthcare Research and Quality (AHRQ). *Recommendations for a National Mass Patient and Evacuee Movement, Regulating, and Tracking System.* Agency for Healthcare Research and Quality; January 2009.

Alexander D. *Principles of Emergency Planning and Management.* Oxford University Press; 2002.

Brangham W. How did Katrina change how we evacuate pets from disaster? *PBS News Hour.* August 29, 2015. https://www.pbs.org/newshour/nation/hurricane-katrina-change-way-evacuate-pets-devastation. Accessed October 10, 2023.

Bring New Orleans Back Commission. *Infrastructure Committee: Levees and Flood Protection Sub-committee.* January 18, 2006. http://www.columbia.edu/itc/journalism/cases/katrina/City%20of%20New%20Orleans/Bring%20New%20Orleans%20Back%20Commission/BNOB%20Infrastructure%20Levees%20Final%20Report%201-18-05.pdf. Accessed May 25, 2023.

Camp Coordination and Camp Management (CCCM) Cluster. *The MEND Guide: Comprehensive Guide for Planning Mass Evacuations in Natural Disasters; Pilot Document.* 2014. https://www.cccmcluster.org/resources/mend-guide. Accessed May 25, 2023.

Centers for Disease Control and Prevention (CDC). *Prevent Illness After a Disaster.* https://www.cdc.gov/disasters/disease/facts.html. Accessed May 25, 2023.

City of Los Angeles. Evacuation functional support annex. In: *City of Los Angeles: Emergency Operations Plan.* October 2020. https://emergency.lacity.gov/sites/g/files/wph1791/files/2022-09/Evacuation%20Annex%20%282020%29.pdf. Accessed May 25, 2023.

Dosa D, Hyer K, Thomas K, et al. To evacuate or shelter in place: implications of universal hurricane evacuation policies on nursing home residents. *J Am Med Dir Assoc.* 2012;13(2):190.e1–e7. doi:10.1016/j.jamda.2011.07.011

Dostal PJ. Vulnerability of urban homebound older adults in disasters: a survey of evacuation preparedness. *Disaster Med Public Health Prep.* 2015;9(3):301–306.

Drevets T. Common injuries people get during disasters. Urban Survival Site. https://urbansurvivalsite.com/common-injuries-disasters/. Accessed May 25, 2023.

Federal Emergency Management Agency (FEMA). Natural hazards. https://hazards.fema.gov/nri/natural-hazards. Accessed May 25, 2023.

Florida Department of Health. Special needs shelters. https://www.floridahealth.gov/programs-and-services/emergency-preparedness-and-response/disaster-response-resources/spns-index.html. Accessed May 25, 2023.

Freedy JR, Simpson WM Jr. Disaster-related physical and mental health: a role for the family physician. *Am Fam Physician.* 2007;75(6):841–846.

Furin MA, Brenner BE. Disaster planning. *Medscape.* July 30, 2018. https://emedicine.medscape.com/article/765495-overview. Accessed May 25, 2023.

Graue J. Normal Fire Department uses tacos to educate on weather lingo (and go viral). WGLT (NPR Network). July 7, 2021. https://www.wglt.org/local-news/2021-07-07/normal-fire-department-uses-tacos-to-educate-on-weather-lingo-and-go-viral. Accessed May 25, 2023.

Internal Displacement Monitoring Centre (iDMC) and Norwegian Refugee Council (NRC). Global estimates 2012: people displaced by disasters. May 2013. https://biotech.law.lsu.edu/blog/global-estimates-2012-may2013.pdf. Accessed May 25, 2023.

Megna M, Tilford A. Pet ownership statistics 2023. *Forbes.* June 21, 2023. https://www.forbes.com/advisor/pet-insurance/pet-ownership-statistics. Accessed October 10, 2023.

National Academies of Sciences, Engineering, and Medicine. *A Safer Future: Reducing the Impacts of Natural Disasters.* National Academies Press; 1991.

Noji EK, Sivertson KT. Injury prevention in natural disasters: a theoretical framework. *Disasters.* 1987;11(4):290–296.

Office of Operations, U.S. Department of Transportation. Evacuating populations with special needs. Federal Highway Administration. https://ops.fhwa.dot.gov/publications/fhwahop09022/sn1_overview.htm. Accessed September 5, 2023.

U.S. Department of Health & Human Services. HHS emPOWER Map. https://empowerprogram.hhs.gov/empowermap. Accessed December 7, 2023.

U.S. Department of Health and Human Services, Administration for Strategic Preparedness and Response. NDMS patient movement program. https://aspr.hhs.gov/NDMS/Pages/patient-mvmt.aspx. Accessed May 25, 2023.

U.S. Department of Homeland Security. Ready.gov: An official website of the U.S. Department of Homeland Security. https://www.ready.gov. Accessed December 7, 2023.

U.S. Department of Transportation Federal Highway Administration. *Evacuating Populations with Special Needs: Routes to Effective Evacuation Planning Primer Series.* U.S. Department of Transportation. April 2009. https://www.hsdl.org/?view&did=35645. Accessed May 25, 2023.

United Nations Climate Change. Climate change leads to more extreme weather, but early warnings save lives. September 1, 2021. https://unfccc.int/news/climate-change-leads-to-more-extreme-weather-but-early-warnings-save-lives. Accessed May 25, 2023.

Waugh WL Jr. Local emergency management in the post-9/11 world. In: Waugh WL Jr, Tierney KT, eds. *Emergency Management: Principles and Practice for Local Government.* 2nd ed. ICMA Press; January 2007.

World Meteorological Organization. Weather-related disasters increase over past 50 years, causing more damage but fewer deaths. August 31, 2021. https://public.wmo.int/en/media/press-release/weather-related-disasters-increase-over-past-50-years-causing-more-damage-fewer. Accessed July 24, 2023.

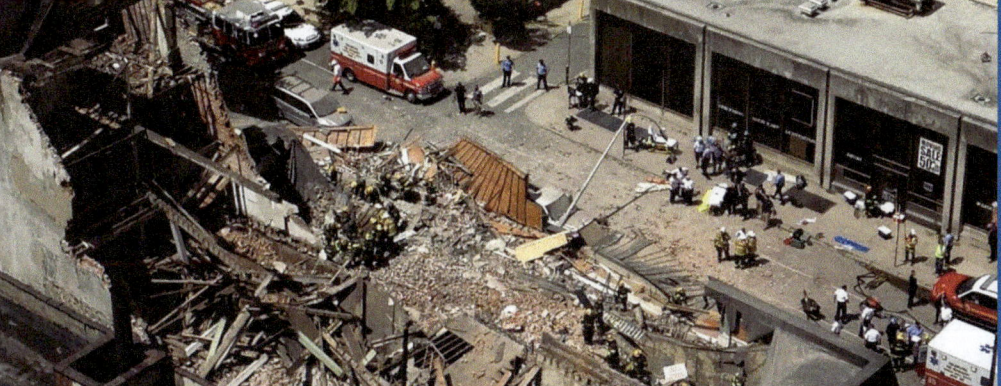

Infectious Diseases and Biologic Disasters

LESSON OBJECTIVES

At the completion of this lesson, you should be able to do the following:

- List the biologic agents that EMS practitioners may encounter.
- Explain the donning and doffing PPE procedure for infectious disease outbreaks or biologic disaster response.
- List the infection control precautions that must be followed for infectious disease outbreaks or biologic disaster response.
- Describe the strategies for ambulance modifications for infectious disease outbreaks or biologic disaster response.

General Considerations

Biologic agents in the form of contagious disease exposure represent a threat to EMS practitioners daily. Exposure can be due to a known or anticipated pathogen in the practitioner's area (e.g., varicella), a new variant of an agent causing an outbreak or a pandemic (e.g., SARS-CoV-2), or a biologic agent that has been weaponized (e.g., smallpox). Preparing for such events increases the complexity of EMS system preparation, requiring appropriate personal protective equipment (PPE), infection control procedures, decontamination of victims, and, possibly, ambulance modification. This section will discuss such aspects of EMS response to a biologic disaster.

Disease Outbreak Terminology

Various terms are used to describe the impact and geographic spread of infectious diseases (**Figure 6-1**). An infectious disease is **endemic** when regularly found within a community at a given baseline (e.g., chickenpox, herpes). An **outbreak** is when there is an increase in the number of infected people in a limited geographic area (e.g., *E. coli*).

An **epidemic** is an infectious disease outbreak leading to an increase in the number of infected people in a larger community or region (bigger area than an outbreak). The disease could be brought in from an outside source, such as a traveler, or it could result from a mutated pathogen that has become more virulent. A **pandemic** is an epidemic that has spread over several countries or continents, usually affecting many people. COVID-19 began as an epidemic and then progressed to a pandemic. The 1918 influenza is another example of a pandemic.

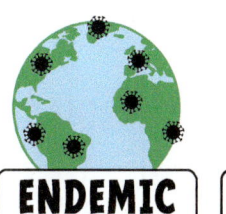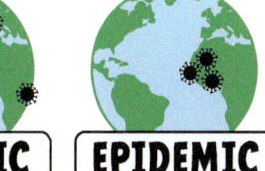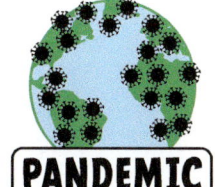

Figure 6-1 Terms used to describe the spread of infectious diseases depend on the impact and geographic prevalence of the disease.
© Ridackan/Shutterstock

Models of Infectious Disease Transmission

General transmission of infectious diseases is due to environmental and animal factors and results from direct and indirect modes of contact (**Figure 6-2**):

- Direct contact is further broken down into person-to-person contact and droplet spread.
- Indirect contact includes airborne, vector-borne, and vehicle-borne modes.

Person-to-person contact, such as kissing, sexual intercourse, other body surface contact, or exchange of body fluids, can transmit certain pathogens between an infectious person (host) and another person. Examples include sexually transmitted infections (STIs), methicillin-resistant *Staphylococcus aureus* (MRSA), and conjunctivitis.

Droplet spread occurs when relatively larger infectious aerosols are generated from actions such as coughing, breathing, or sneezing. These droplets often travel short distances (a few feet), so close proximity to the host is necessary for the disease to spread. *Neisseria meningitidis*, influenza virus, and *Bordetella pertussis* are common droplet-spread pathogens.

Airborne transmission occurs when very small droplets are expelled from an infected respiratory tract. These droplets are small enough to remain airborne in air currents for long periods, during which another person may inhale them. Tuberculosis, measles, and COVID-19 are examples of diseases spread by airborne transmission.

Vector-borne transmission of an infectious organism occurs when it is introduced to a human by an intermediate carrier or reservoir. Examples of vector-borne transmission include West Nile virus, which is transmitted by the bite of a mosquito, and Lyme disease, which is transmitted by the bite of a blacklegged tick.

Items, including biologic materials, that are not necessarily infectious but may transmit infectious pathogens

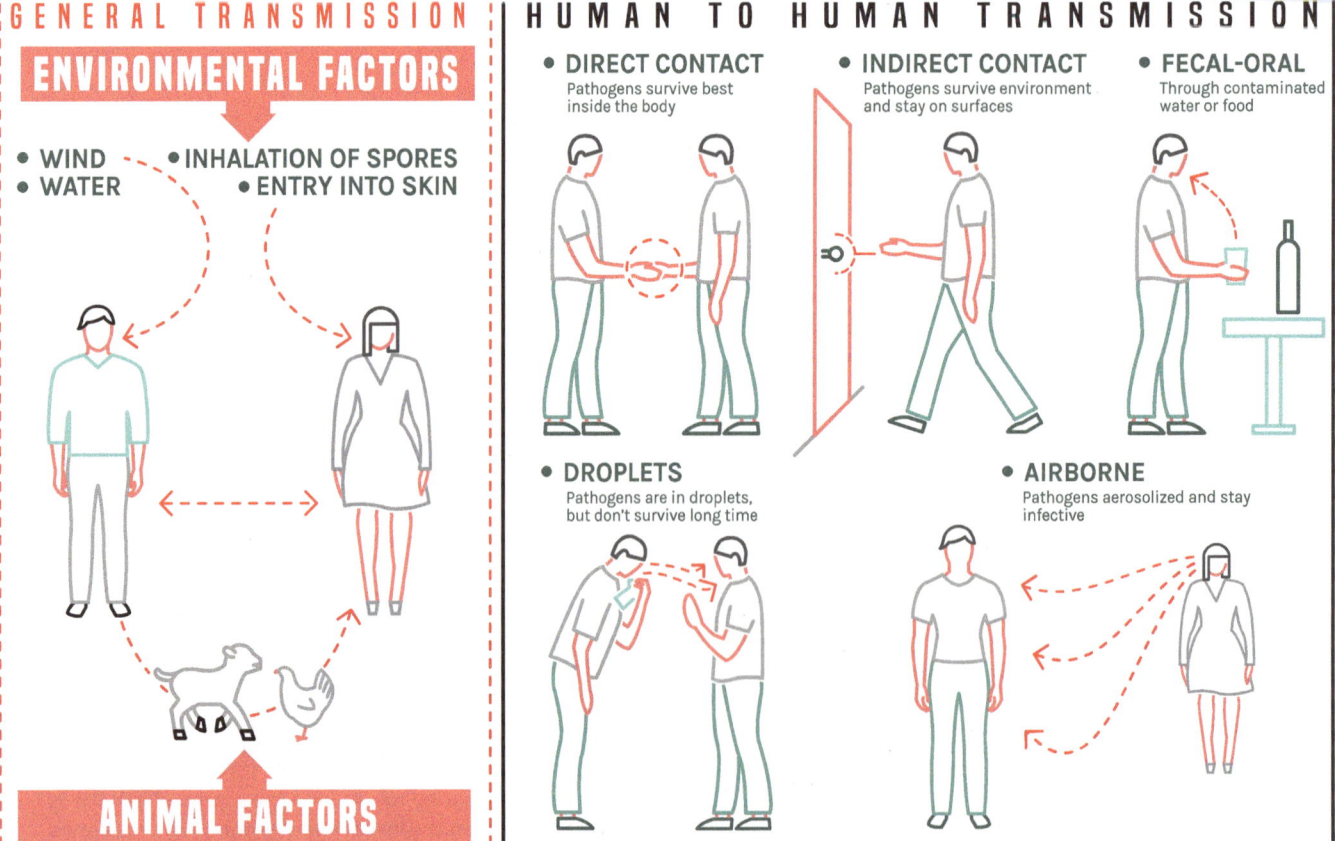

Figure 6-2 Models of infectious disease transmission.

are considered vehicles. Vehicles may carry a pathogen or may be a reservoir for an infectious agent. **Vehicle-borne transmission** examples include drinking water contaminated with *Escherichia coli* and contaminated foods containing *Salmonella* bacteria. Fomites are inanimate objects (e.g., doorknobs, surgical equipment) that may transmit illness.

Controlling Infectious Disease Transmission

Source control is the principle of controlling the spread of potentially infectious material at the source. If patients have an infectious disease that could be transmitted via droplet or airborne routes, EMS practitioners should offer them a face mask if they are not currently wearing one and can tolerate it. Masks should be placed on the patients upon initial contact and remain in place until cleared by incident command or when the patient is transported. Additionally, medical face masks (e.g., surgical masks) or cloth masks should be provided to those without masks based on available supplies.

Face masks should not be placed on certain patients, including patients younger than 2 years of age and patients who have trouble breathing, are unconscious, are incapacitated, or are unable to remove the mask without assistance. Source control can also be achieved with a filter on an endotracheal tube, nebulizer, ventilator circuit, continuous positive airway pressure (CPAP) or bilevel positive airway pressure (BPAP) mask, or bag-valve mask device.

Standard precautions involve treating all blood and body fluid as potentially infectious. Wear gloves when contact with body fluids or potential for infectious disease is anticipated. Wear a gown, mask, and goggles or face shield when performing procedures with an increased risk of exposure to blood or other potentially infectious materials (**Figure 6-3**).

> ## When *Not* to Place Medical Face Masks
>
> - Patients younger than 2 years
> - Patients who have trouble breathing
> - Unconscious patients
> - Incapacitated patients
> - Patients who are unable to remove the mask without assistance

Contact precautions are recommended to reduce the likelihood of transmission of microorganisms by direct or indirect contact and include gloves and a gown (**Figure 6-4**). Contact precautions are required to prevent the spread of the herpes simplex or zoster virus, viral conjunctivitis, MRSA, and scabies. Strict contact precautions are needed against pathogens that cause bubonic plagues or viral hemorrhagic fevers, such as Marburg or Ebola, *as long as the patient does not have pulmonary symptoms or profuse vomiting and diarrhea*, in which case airborne precautions should also be taken.

Droplet precautions are recommended to reduce the likelihood of microorganisms transmitted by large droplets expelled by an infected person during talking, sneezing, or coughing or during routine procedures such as suctioning. These droplets infect by landing on the exposed mucous membranes of the eyes, nose, and mouth. Because the large droplets do not remain suspended in air, contact must be in close proximity, usually defined as 3 feet or less.

Droplet precautions include the contact precautions of gloves and gown and additional eye protection and a surgical mask. Because the droplets do not remain

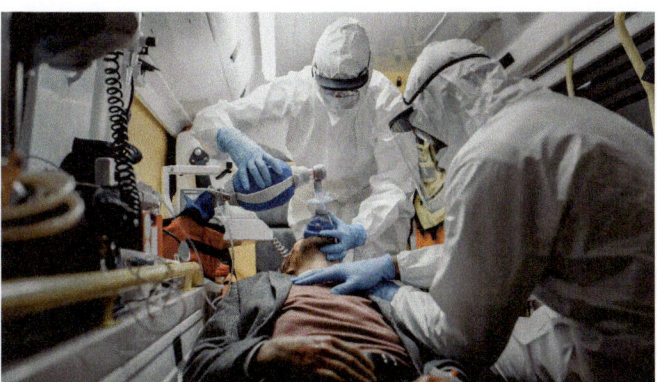

Figure 6-3 Standard precautions help prevent the spread of infectious disease.
© Gorodenkoff/Shutterstock

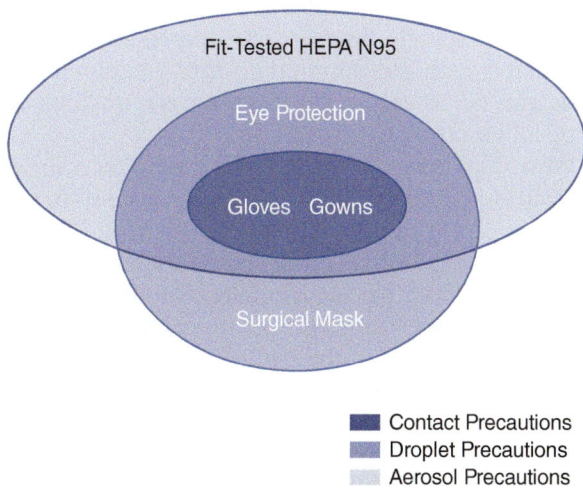

Figure 6-4 Contact, droplet, and aerosol precautions.
© National Association of Emergency Medical Technicians (NAEMT)

suspended in the air, no additional respiratory protection or air filtration is required. Typically encountered organisms that require droplet precautions include the influenza virus, *Mycoplasma pneumoniae*, and invasive *Haemophilus influenzae* or *Neisseria meningitidis*, which can cause sepsis or meningitis. The microorganism that causes pneumonic plague is an example of a droplet-borne bacteria that could be encountered due to a bioterrorist event.

Aerosol precautions are recommended to reduce the likelihood of transmission of microorganisms by the airborne route. Some organisms can become suspended in the air attached to small droplet nuclei (less than 5 µm) or attached to dust particles. In this case, microorganisms can become widely dispersed by air currents immediately around the source or more distant from the source, depending on environmental conditions. To avoid such dispersion, once the pathogen is confirmed, these patients are kept in negative-pressure isolation rooms in a hospital in which the exhaust ventilation can be filtered.

Aerosol precautions include gloves, gown, eye protection, and a fit-tested high-efficiency particulate air (HEPA) filter mask, such as the N95. Examples of illnesses typically encountered requiring aerosol precautions include tuberculosis, measles, chickenpox, and SARS and its variants, including SARS-CoV-2. Smallpox and viral hemorrhagic fever with pulmonary symptoms are examples of illnesses requiring aerosol precautions that could be related to a bioterrorist event.

Personal Protective Equipment (PPE)

Fit Testing PPE

PPE is fit tested to verify the sufficiency of the respirator seal on the user's face. In the event of an infectious disease and biologic disaster, EMS practitioners should be prepared with the appropriate-fitting equipment. Fit testing can be accomplished in two ways: qualitative fit testing and quantitative fit testing.

With qualitative fit testing, the respirator user performs various exercises while exposed to a solution to see if the user can taste it (either sweet or bitter). If the respirator user does not taste the solution after completing the fit test, the user has an adequate seal (fit test passed). If the respirator user tastes the solution during the fit test, the user has a breach in the seal (fit test failed).

With quantitative fit testing, the respirator is attached to a machine that guides the user through various exercises. During the exercises, the machine measures the amount of leak in the seal. Based on the level of the leak, the machine will designate the respirator's fit as a pass or a fail.

Types of PPE

PPE provides a line of defense against infectious pathogens (**Table 6-1**). Appropriate PPE must be worn when responding to infectious diseases or biologic disasters (**Figure 6-5**). This ranges from gloves for a standard patient encounter to a fully encapsulated suit with **self-contained breathing apparatus (SCBA)**, depending on the specific agent involved, proximity to the threat, and the level of training and role of the responder.

Level A PPE offers the highest level of respiratory and skin protection. It is most often used in the hot zone. However, it takes a considerable amount of time to don, thus delaying the practitioner's ability to access and help patients. It makes manual tasks difficult to perform, requires significant training and experience, and puts the wearer at risk for heat stress and physical exhaustion. Furthermore, it can make communication between EMS

Table 6-1 Types of PPE

Types of PPE	Description
Level A	Respiratory tract protected by a self-contained breathing apparatus (SCBA) or **supplied air respirator (SAR)** delivering air to the EMS practitioner with positive pressure + A chemical-resistant barrier completely encapsulates the wearer, protecting the skin and mucous membranes
Level B	Respiratory tract protected in the same manner as in level A protection, with positive-pressure–supplied air + Nonencapsulated chemical-resistant garments (suit, gloves, and boots) provide splash protection only
Level C	Respiratory tract protected by an air-purifying respirator (APR) + Skin protection same as for level B
Level D	Standard work clothes (i.e., standard uniform for the emergency responder) and may also include gown, gloves, and surgical mask

© National Association of Emergency Medical Technicians (NAEMT)

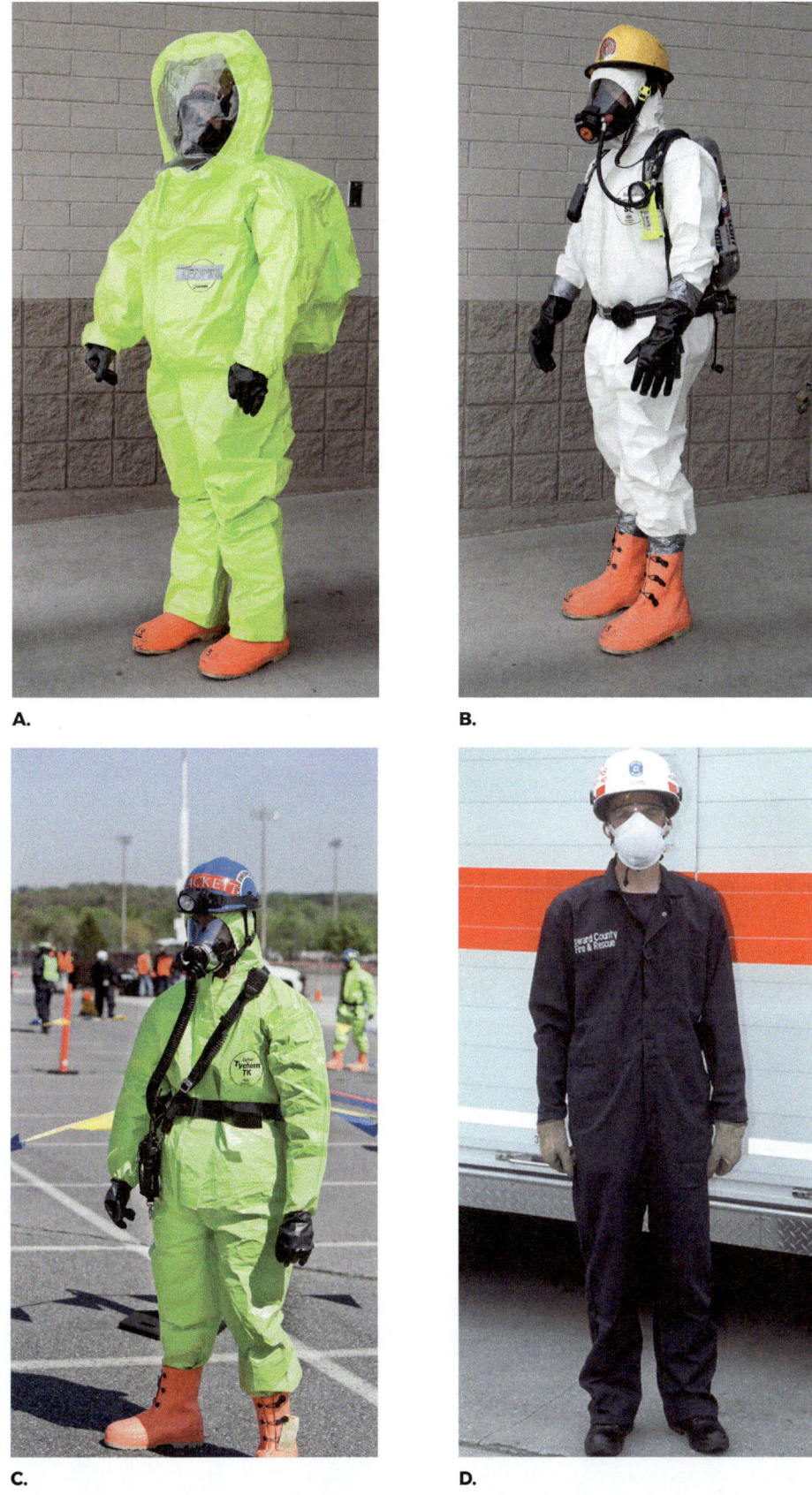

Figure 6-5 Personal protective equipment. **A.** Level A. **B.** Level B. **C.** Level C. **D.** Level D.

A-C: Courtesy of Rick Brady; D: © Jones & Bartlett Learning. Courtesy of MIEMSS

practitioners and victims very difficult. *Note: The available air supply, the buildup of heat and humidity within the enclosed suit, and specific agency work/rest protocols limit the time a practitioner can spend in level A PPE.*

Level B PPE affords the highest respiratory protection, with a lower skin protection level than level A PPE. Like level A protection, level B protection takes time to don and doff, and work time within the suit is limited. **Level C PPE** offers less respiratory protection than level B but similar skin protection. **Level D PPE** represents standard work clothes (i.e., a standard uniform for EMS practitioners) and may include a gown, gloves, and surgical

mask. Level D provides minimal respiratory protection and minimal skin protection.

Donning and Doffing PPE

Putting on PPE (called donning PPE) is done in a certain order to ensure that the user is adequately protected (**Figure 6-6**).

Taking PPE off (called doffing PPE) is done in a certain order to ensure that wearers do not inadvertently contaminate themselves during the process (**Figure 6-7**). *EMS practitioners must use safe work practices to protect*

SEQUENCE FOR PUTTING ON PERSONAL PROTECTIVE EQUIPMENT (PPE)

The type of PPE used will vary based on the level of precautions required, such as standard and contact, droplet or airborne infection isolation precautions. The procedure for putting on and removing PPE should be tailored to the specific type of PPE.

1. GOWN

- Fully cover torso from neck to knees, arms to end of wrists, and wrap around the back
- Fasten in back of neck and waist

2. MASK OR RESPIRATOR

- Secure ties or elastic bands at middle of head and neck
- Fit flexible band to nose bridge
- Fit snug to face and below chin
- Fit-check respirator

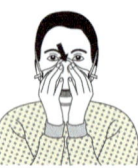

3. GOGGLES OR FACE SHIELD

- Place over face and eyes and adjust to fit

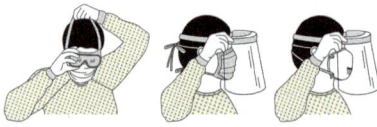

4. GLOVES

- Extend to cover wrist of isolation gown

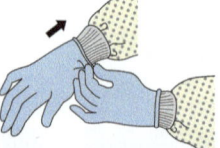

USE SAFE WORK PRACTICES TO PROTECT YOURSELF AND LIMIT THE SPREAD OF CONTAMINATION

- Keep hands away from face
- Limit surfaces touched
- Change gloves when torn or heavily contaminated
- Perform hand hygiene

Figure 6-6 Procedure for donning PPE.

Courtesy of the Centers for Disease Control and Prevention. Reference to specific commercial products, manufacturers, companies, or trademarks does not constitute its endorsement or recommendation by the U.S. Government, Department of Health and Human Services, or Centers for Disease Control and Prevention. Available free of charge at https://www.cdc.gov/hai/pdfs/ppe/PPE-Sequence.pdf.

HOW TO SAFELY REMOVE PERSONAL PROTECTIVE EQUIPMENT (PPE) EXAMPLE 1

There are a variety of ways to safely remove PPE without contaminating your clothing, skin, or mucous membranes with potentially infectious materials. Here is one example. **Remove all PPE before exiting the patient room** except a respirator, if worn. Remove the respirator **after** leaving the patient room and closing the door. Remove PPE in the following sequence:

1. GLOVES

- Outside of gloves are contaminated!
- If your hands get contaminated during glove removal, immediately wash your hands or use an alcohol-based hand sanitizer
- Using a gloved hand, grasp the palm area of the other gloved hand and peel off first glove
- Hold removed glove in gloved hand
- Slide fingers of ungloved hand under remaining glove at wrist and peel off second glove over first glove
- Discard gloves in a waste container

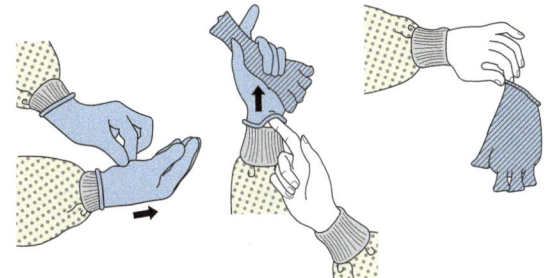

2. GOGGLES OR FACE SHIELD

- Outside of goggles or face shield are contaminated!
- If your hands get contaminated during goggle or face shield removal, immediately wash your hands or use an alcohol-based hand sanitizer
- Remove goggles or face shield from the back by lifting head band or ear pieces
- If the item is reusable, place in designated receptacle for reprocessing. Otherwise, discard in a waste container

3. GOWN

- Gown front and sleeves are contaminated!
- If your hands get contaminated during gown removal, immediately wash your hands or use an alcohol-based hand sanitizer
- Unfasten gown ties, taking care that sleeves don't contact your body when reaching for ties
- Pull gown away from neck and shoulders, touching inside of gown only
- Turn gown inside out
- Fold or roll into a bundle and discard in a waste container

4. MASK OR RESPIRATOR

- Front of mask/respirator is contaminated — DO NOT TOUCH!
- If your hands get contaminated during mask/respirator removal, immediately wash your hands or use an alcohol-based hand sanitizer
- Grasp bottom ties or elastics of the mask/respirator, then the ones at the top, and remove without touching the front
- Discard in a waste container

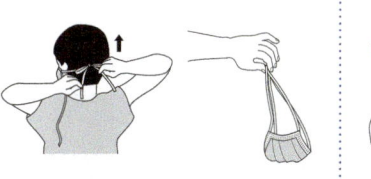
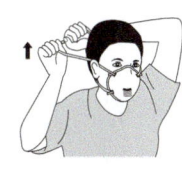

5. WASH HANDS OR USE AN ALCOHOL-BASED HAND SANITIZER IMMEDIATELY AFTER REMOVING ALL PPE

OR

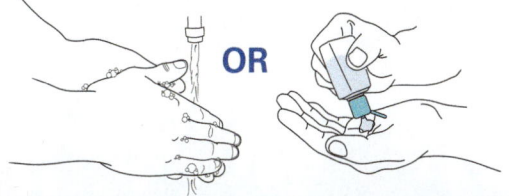

PERFORM HAND HYGIENE BETWEEN STEPS IF HANDS BECOME CONTAMINATED AND IMMEDIATELY AFTER REMOVING ALL PPE

Figure 6-7 Procedure for doffing PPE.

Courtesy of the Centers for Disease Control and Prevention. Reference to specific commercial products, manufacturers, companies, or trademarks does not constitute its endorsement or recommendation by the U.S. Government, Department of Health and Human Services, or Centers for Disease Control and Prevention. Available free of charge at https://www.cdc.gov/hai/pdfs/ppe/PPE-Sequence.pdf.

themselves and limit the spread of contamination. In addition to the doffing procedure described in Figure 6-7, practitioners should follow these guidelines:

- Remove PPE at the doorway or in an anteroom of the involved room.
- Remove the respirator after leaving the contaminated room and closing the door.
- Once PPE is removed, wash your hands.
- If your hands become contaminated during any step of removing PPE, immediately wash them or use an alcohol-based sanitizer.

Note: Contamination risk to EMS practitioners is very high during the doffing process. If possible, a safety monitor should be used.

Decontamination

Various **decontamination** strategies can be used to limit the spread of infectious organisms based on the specific situation:

- Decontamination of clothing by washing with soap and water
- Decontamination of equipment using a 0.1% sodium hypochlorite bleach solution (1:1,000 diluted bleach solution)
- Autoclaving or high-level disinfection of reusable medical equipment
- Careful decontamination of ambulance and equipment with disinfectant wipes, ultraviolet radiation, or disinfectant misting (dry fogging) (**Figure 6-8**)
- Cleaning of environmental surfaces with a detergent/disinfectant product registered by the Environmental Protection Agency (EPA)

Ambulance Modification

Ambulance modification may be necessary when transporting highly infectious patients, as in the case of viral hemorrhagic fevers such as "wet" Ebola, pneumonic plague, Middle East respiratory syndrome (MERS), smallpox, or measles. Modifications could involve the following:

- Isolating the driver compartment
- Covering all equipment/surfaces within the patient compartment (**Figure 6-9**)
- Isolating patients in a contamination-limiting suit or capsule

Bioterrorism and Disasters

Bioterrorism is when biologic agents are used on the human population, animals, and crops to cause harm or invoke fear. This section will discuss what makes a biologic agent a bioterrorism agent and explore the Centers for Disease Control and Prevention (CDC) risk categories for these agents.

Bioterrorism incidents typically do not call attention to themselves. There is often no discrete incident scene, dramatic explosion, blazing cone of fire, or hail of shrapnel. The insidious or gradual onset of symptoms associated with biologic agents makes them all the more threatening because, during the pathogen's incubation, many people in a wide geographic area may become ill before health officials recognize a pattern of illness. Public health authorities then notice a higher-than-expected

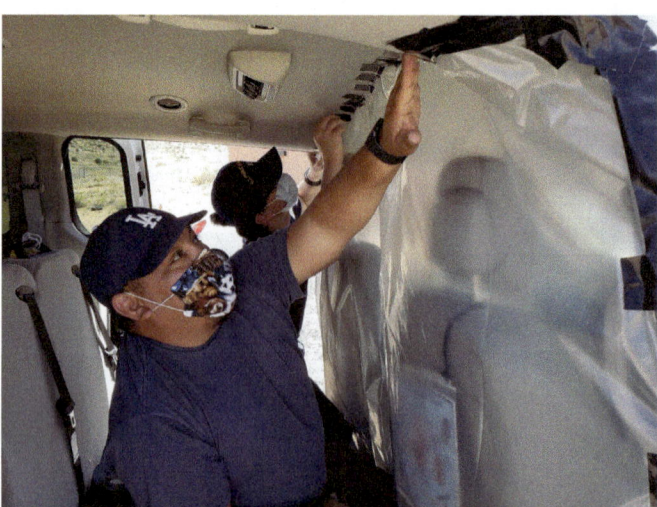

Figure 6-9 Ambulance modification, such as covering surfaces/equipment with plastic, may be necessary when transporting highly infectious patients.

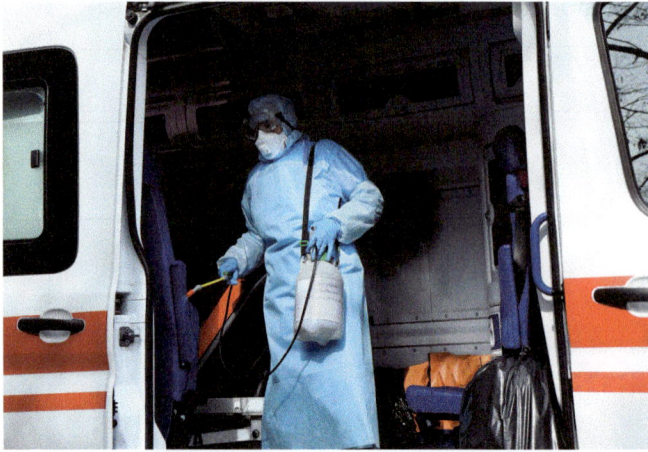

Figure 6-8 Disinfectant misting may be used to decontaminate the ambulance.

incidence of certain signs and symptoms or similar chief complaints within a given geographic area. Perhaps they are tipped off by an unusual disease presentation, a heavy load of cases within a circumscribed area, or reports of unusual routes of exposure.

What Makes a Biologic Agent a Bioterrorism Agent?

The following are common characteristics of bioterrorism agents:

- Delivery using simple technology
- Capability for delivery from a source upwind from their target (such as an airplane) to infect a large population
- Ability to cause widespread panic, fear, infection, and disease

Bioterrorism agents have a number of possible routes of transmission:

- Aerosolized agents (most likely)
- Contaminated food or water supply
- Letters or packages
- Infected animal used as a vector
- Human-to-human contact

CDC Risk Categories for Bioterrorism Agents

An intentional terrorist act might include delivery of a biologic agent, such as aerosolized spores, water supply contaminated with live organisms, or an aerosolized biologic toxin, with the potential to cause disease or illness.

The CDC categorizes bioterrorism agents by priority level, based on their potential impact (**Table 6-2**).

Category A bioterrorism agents pose the highest risk to national security and public health. They can be easily disseminated or transmitted from person to person, resulting in high mortality rates. They have the potential for a major public health impact, might cause social disruption, and require special action for public health preparedness. Examples include *Bacillus anthracis*, *Clostridium botulinum* (botulinum toxins), *Yersinia pestis*, variola major, *Francisella tularensis*, filoviruses (Ebola, Marburg), and arenaviruses (Lassa fever, Machupo). Responding to a threat involving Category A bioterrorism agents would require level A PPE.

Category A bioterrorism agents have been weaponized by countries and terrorist organizations and have the potential to cause catastrophe. Consider the following hypothetical scenarios. A release of 220 pounds of anthrax spores over Washington, DC, could result in 130,000 to 3 million deaths! A release of 110 pounds of aerosolized *Y. pestis* over a city of 5 million would result in 150,000 cases of pneumonic plague and 36,000 deaths. A terrorist point-source delivery of botulinum aerosol could incapacitate or kill 10% of persons as far as 0.3 mile downwind.

Category B bioterrorism agents are moderately easy to disseminate, result in moderate morbidity and low mortality rates, and require specific enhancements of the CDC's diagnostic capacity and disease surveillance. Examples include water safety threats (e.g., *V. cholerae*, *Cryptosporidium parvum*), food safety threats (e.g., *Salmonella* spp., *E. coli* O157:H7), toxins (e.g., ricin, staphylococcal enterotoxin B), alphaviruses (Venezuelan equine

Table 6-2 Categories of Bioterrorism Agents		
Category A	**Category B**	**Category C**
Anthrax	Brucellosis	Emerging infectious diseases
Botulism	*Clostridium perfringens*	■ Hantavirus
Plague	Food safety threats (e.g., *Salmonella* species, *Escherichia coli*)	■ Nipah virus
Smallpox	Glanders	
Tularemia	Melioidosis	
Viral hemorrhagic fevers	Psittacosis	
■ Filoviruses	Q fever	
■ Arenaviruses	Ricin toxin	
	Staphylococcal enterotoxin B	
	Typhus fever	
	Viral encephalitis	
	Water safety threats (e.g., *Vibrio cholerae*, *Cryptosporidium parvum*)	

Modified from Centers for Disease Control and Prevention. Bioterrorism agents/diseases. Accessed October 2, 2023. https://emergency.cdc.gov/agent/agentlist-category.asp

encephalitis, Eastern equine encephalitis, Western equine encephalitis), *Brucella* spp., and *Coxiella burnetii*.

Category C bioterrorism agents are emerging pathogens that pose a risk due to the potential to be engineered for mass dissemination, availability, ease of production and dissemination, high morbidity and mortality rates, and potential for major health impact. Examples include Nipah virus and hantavirus.

EMS Response: Infectious Diseases and Biologic Disasters

In many situations, unless a person or group claims responsibility for a bioterrorism attack, it may not be immediately detected as such until clusters of cases appear. Public health surveillance becomes extremely crucial in these circumstances. This section will discuss aspects of EMS response to infectious diseases and biologic disasters.

EMS Practitioners and Bioterrorism

EMS practitioners can experience bioterrorism in two ways (**Figure 6-10**). The first way could involve the overt release of a material that is either identified as or thought to be a biologic agent. The anthrax hoaxes of 1998 and 1999 and the anthrax letters of 2001 are good examples. Practitioners responded on countless occasions to individuals covered in "white powder" or suspected anthrax.

The second way could be responding to a patient who is a victim of a bioterrorist event. Perhaps the patient inhaled anthrax spores after a covert attack at work and now, several days later, is manifesting signs of pulmonary anthrax. Perhaps a terrorist has self-inoculated

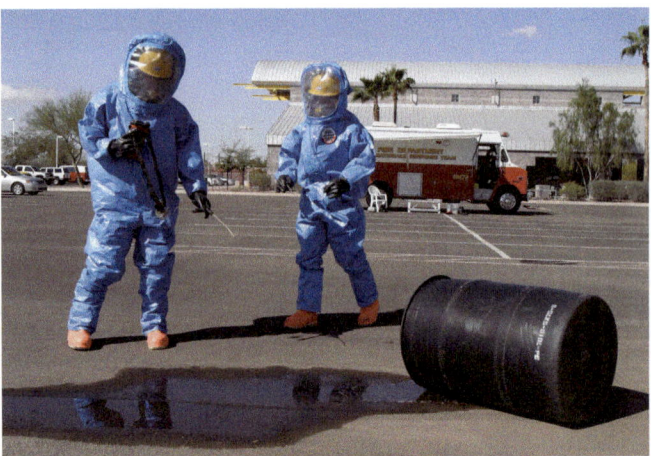

Figure 6-10 EMS practitioners and bioterrorism.
© Jones and Bartlett Publishers. Courtesy of MIEMSS.

with smallpox, and you are summoned to assist a person with a suspicious rash.

General EMS Response: Concentrated Biohazard Agent vs. Infected Patient

The nature of the threat in the event of a concentrated biohazard agent release is usually unknown, and precautions for personal safety should always be paramount. These incidents must be treated as a **weapon of mass destruction (WMD)** incident until proven otherwise. If the suspicious substance is a concentrated aerosol of an infectious organism or toxin, PPE appropriate for the biologic agent is required. You must also follow local decontamination protocols.

When EMS practitioners respond to a victim of a bioterrorist event or an infected patient, knowledge of proper infection control procedures and the proper donning and removal of PPE appropriate for the biohazard can help to ensure personal and public safety. The type of PPE used will vary based on the required precautions (e.g., standard precautions, contact precautions, droplet precautions, aerosol precautions). Decontamination of the patient in this scenario is unnecessary, but source control remains important.

How Is Biologic Triage Different?

Disaster, or mass-casualty, triage, as discussed in Chapter 3, is a process of sorting casualties into the order of priority based on their injuries. It requires a prompt assessment by responding practitioners, who often must perform lifesaving interventions on site.

Biologic emergencies will likely not present immediately, and there is not always a specific incident scene. A surge of ill patients is likely (similar to early in the COVID-19 pandemic). Moreover, when a pathogen is easily transmitted, EMS practitioners are more likely to see deaths from infectious diseases than from traumatic events, and this risk is ongoing (as opposed to a one-time traumatic event). The lifesaving interventions of mass-casualty triage do not apply in biologic emergencies. That is, you are less likely to have patients with penetrating or blunt trauma resulting in life-threatening external hemorrhage or tension pneumothorax.

Biologic triage aims to help control transmission, minimize the spread of illness, and assist with resource allocation and prioritization. Triage criteria for infectious diseases may include clinical signs and symptoms related to the suspected pathogen and could divide the patients into the following categories: susceptible but not exposed, exposed but not yet infectious, infectious, removed by death or recovery, and protected by vaccination or prophylactic medication.

Specific Steps to Prevent Infection

- Utilize the information provided by dispatch to identify patients with symptoms of potentially highly infectious diseases.
- Maintain a heightened awareness of the potential of interacting with patients with new and drug-resistant organisms.
- Limit the number of personnel who have initial contact with patients.
  - Conduct the "view from the door" to determine the need for multiple practitioners.
  - Should such an impression not be clear, only the minimum number of EMS practitioners necessary or a triage officer in the appropriate PPE should make contact and conduct patient triage.
- Obtain a thorough travel history for the past month.
  - Ask patients about any recent domestic and international travel.
  - Ask patients about potential sources of exposure.
- Wear the appropriate level of PPE based on the mode of transmission of the suspected agent (**Figure 6-11**).
- Provide surgical masks to all patients with symptoms of a respiratory illness who can tolerate it.
- Conduct active surveillance for infected sores, ulcers, lesions, and drainage that may or may not be contained by dressings.
- Use contact precautions during close patient contact.
- Use impermeable barrier sheets to cover patients with excessive secretions to help minimize contamination of surfaces and protect EMS practitioners.
- Confirm that the hospital or other receiving facilities have been notified of the possibility of an infectious disease or biologic disaster.
- Perform thorough cleaning of all equipment and the environmental surfaces that had contact with the patients.

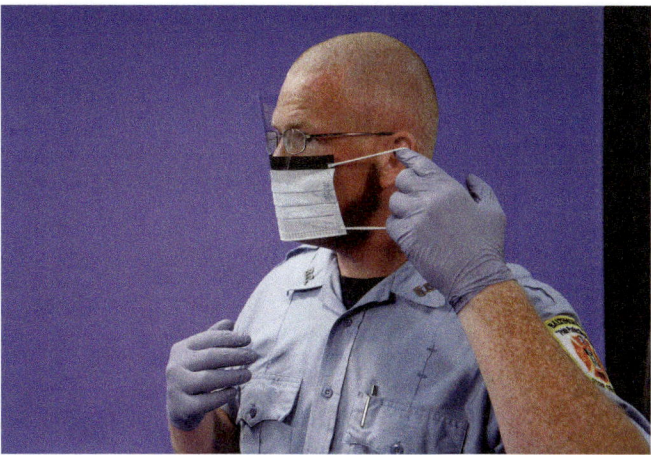

Figure 6-11 PPE during a biologic emergency is based on the mode of transmission of the suspect agent.
© Jones & Bartlett Learning. Courtesy of MIEMSS.

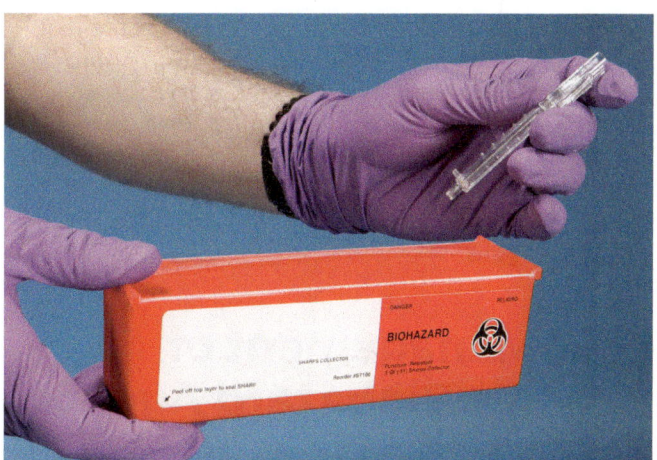

Figure 6-12 Sharps must be disposed of in the appropriate container.
© Jones & Bartlett Learning. Courtesy of MIEMSS.

- Ensure that all disinfecting agents are approved for use against the suspected pathogen.
- Pay attention to the surface contact time (the time that a disinfectant needs to be in contact with the surface to "kill" the pathogen).
- Many methods are available to decontaminate ambulances and equipment, including UV radiation, misting (dry fogging), and disinfectant wipes.
- Follow all manufacturers' recommendations when disinfecting your ambulance and equipment.

Other important considerations:

- Use an engineered needle system and proper sharps disposal (**Figure 6-12**).

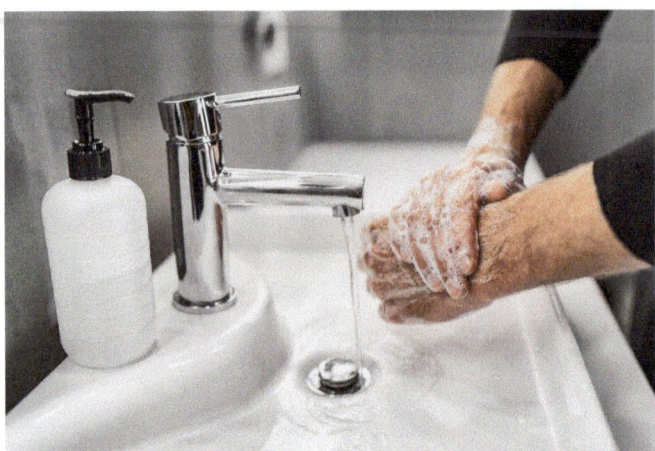

Figure 6-13 EMS personnel must be diligent in performing proper hand hygiene.

© Maridav/Shutterstock

- Self-occluding IV catheters could reduce potential blood exposure.
- Diligently practice proper hand hygiene (**Figure 6-13**).
- If you suspect that patients may have encountered a new or resistant organism, follow your local infection control plan and make appropriate notifications.

EMS Management of Specific Biohazard Agents

Anthrax

Anthrax is an acute infectious disease caused by the gram-positive, spore-forming bacterium *B. anthracis*. The most common route of entry is direct skin contact and absorption of spores, which causes a localized red, itchy ulcer (cutaneous anthrax). Although less common, anthrax can also cause inhalational and gastrointestinal (GI) disease through those routes of exposure.

Within 2 weeks of direct contact with anthrax spores, the skin begins to necrose and a black eschar forms. Anthrax spores that are inhaled may initially cause apparently benign symptoms similar to those of the common cold. In the early prodromal stage, the patient complains of a nonproductive cough, fever, chills, and nausea. After a few days, symptoms improve, followed by a rapidly deteriorating course of high fever, cyanosis, shock, diaphoresis, and severe respiratory distress. Before the 2001 anthrax attacks, mortality from inhalational anthrax was thought to be 90%, but outcomes from those incidents suggest that with early antibiotic therapy and critical care services mortality could be significantly lower.

In the prehospital setting, supportive care with supplemental oxygen, IV therapy for fluid replacement, and application of dry, sterile dressing to wounds is appropriate. You must notify the receiving facility of the exposure. Emergency decontamination is not necessary unless the exposure has just occurred. You are at risk only if you have direct contact with lesions. Inhalation and GI exposure cannot infect others.

Anthrax spores are extremely difficult to destroy and can be easily transported on victims' skin or clothes, presenting an infectious hazard to practitioners. Victims of known or suspected anthrax releases (e.g., letters containing suspicious white powders) should be decontaminated on scene by responders wearing level A PPE to avoid contamination of transport equipment or infection of practitioners by anthrax spores carried on victims' skin or clothes.

Prophylaxis with antibiotics is required only for individuals exposed to spores. Local public health officials will determine the appropriate antibiotic and length of prophylactic treatment. The latest recommendations suggest 60 days of therapy with oral ciprofloxacin or doxycycline and postexposure vaccination.

An anthrax vaccine does exist, and an immunization program for U.S. military forces was instituted in 1998. The current regimen requires a series of six initial shots and annual boosters. It is currently recommended only for military personnel and laboratory and industrial workers at high risk for spore exposure. The CDC has purchased tens of thousands of doses of the anthrax vaccine for the Strategic National Stockpile that would be made available to emergency responders in case of an anthrax incident with risk of exposure.

Plague

Y. pestis is the bacterium that causes plague, which includes pneumonic, bubonic, and septicemic plagues. In pneumonic plague, *Y. pestis* infects the lungs. In bioterrorist attacks, transmission occurs by breathing in aerosolized bacteria. It is also spread person to person by respiratory droplets. This requires close contact with the person or animal infected. In bubonic plague, transmission occurs through the bites of fleas from rodents such as mice, groundhogs, squirrels, and chipmunks. Septicemic plague occurs through pneumonic or bubonic plague complications when bacteria multiply in the blood, leading to septic shock.

Symptoms of pneumonic plague include difficulty breathing, productive cough, bloody sputum, and an associated complaint of chest pain. These symptoms lead to septicemic plague, causing respiratory and cardiovascular collapse if not treated. In bubonic plague, patients have enlarged lymph nodes, altered mentation, agitation, anuria, tachycardia, and hypotension. Untreated bubonic plague can progress to septicemic plague, with symptoms including nausea, vomiting, diarrhea, necrotic skin lesions, and gangrene.

Plague victims are treated in the field with supportive therapy. Communication with the receiving facility is vital before arrival to ensure that the pneumonic plague patient can be properly isolated in the emergency department (ED) and that staff are prepared with the appropriate PPE. Asking the patient to wear a surgical mask, if tolerated, may decrease the likelihood of secondary transmission.

Everyone who has come into contact with the patient should also be evaluated for symptoms. Initiate routine supportive medical care and screen for severe sepsis or septic shock signs. Early intervention with antibiotics and antimicrobial agents is appropriate. Ciprofloxacin, gentamicin, or doxycycline are all options to treat active disease. Appropriate PPE and respiratory precautions, including N95 respirators, should be used to avoid contact with airborne droplets.

Decontamination of the vehicle and equipment is similar to that required after transporting any patient with a communicable disease. Contact surfaces should be wiped down with disinfectant approved by the EPA or a 0.1% sodium hypochlorite bleach solution. No evidence suggests that *Y. pestis* poses a long-term environmental threat after the dissolution of the primary aerosol. The organism is sensitive to heat and sunlight and does not last long outside the living host. *Y. pestis* does not form spores.

Smallpox

Smallpox is also known as variola major and variola minor, depending on the severity of the illness. This naturally occurring viral disease was eradicated in 1977 but still exists in at least two laboratories—Russia's Institute of Virus Preparations and the CDC. It was alleged that the Soviet government began a program in 1980 to produce large quantities of smallpox virus for use in bombs and missiles and to develop more virulent strains of the virus for military purposes. There is also concern that the smallpox virus may have changed hands after the dissolution of the Soviet Union.

The smallpox virus infects its victim by entering the mucous membranes of the oropharynx or respiratory mucosa. After a 12- to 14-day incubation period, the patient develops fever, malaise, headache, and backache. The patient then develops a maculopapular rash that starts on the oral mucosa and quickly progresses to a generalized skin rash with characteristic round, tense vesicles, and pustules. The rash tends to affect the head and extremities more densely than the trunk (centrifugal), with the stage of the lesions appearing uniform; as a memory aid, think *smallpox = same* (**Figure 6-14**). This

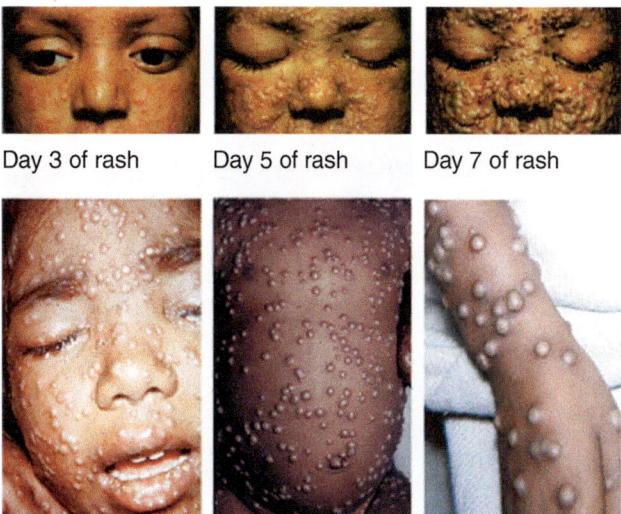

Day 3 of rash   Day 5 of rash   Day 7 of rash

On any part of the body, all lesions are in the same stage of development.

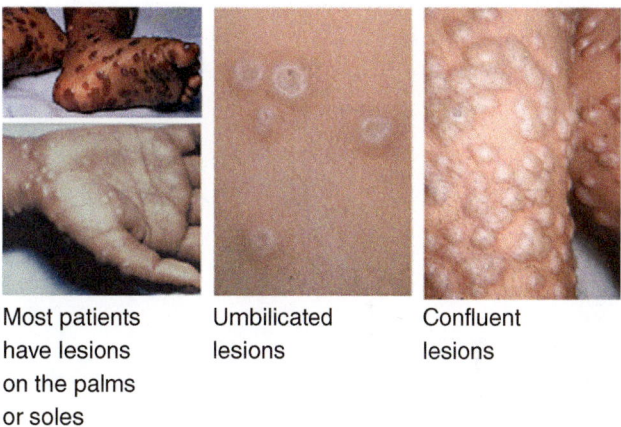

Most patients have lesions on the palms or soles   Umbilicated lesions   Confluent lesions

Figure 6-14 Smallpox presentation.
Courtesy of the Centers for Disease Control and Prevention

presentation distinguishes smallpox from varicella, or chickenpox, which begins on and is denser on the trunk (centripetal) and has lesions at various stages of development (new lesions appear with older, crusted lesions); think *varicella = various* (**Figure 6-15**). Mortality from naturally occurring smallpox was approximately 30%. Little is known about the natural course of the disease in immunocompromised patients, such as those with human immunodeficiency virus (HIV).

Smallpox is a contagious disease primarily spread by droplet nuclei projected from the oropharynx of infected patients and by direct contact. Contaminated clothing and bed linens can (and have been used to) spread the virus. Patients are contagious beginning slightly before the onset of the rash, although this might not always be obvious if the rash is subtle in the oropharynx. When managing a patient with smallpox,

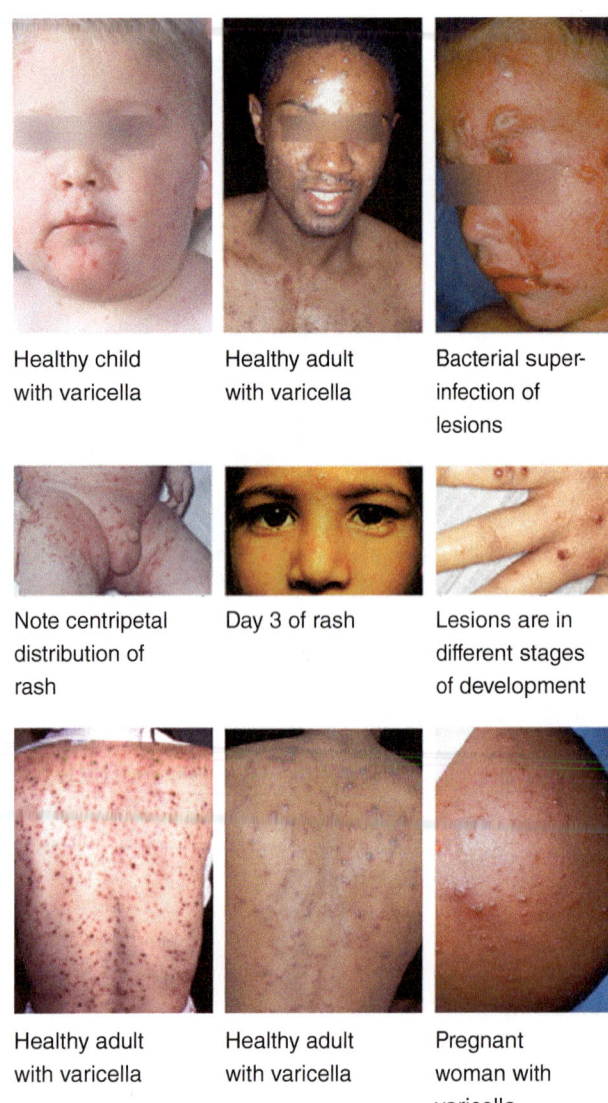

Healthy child with varicella

Healthy adult with varicella

Bacterial super-infection of lesions

Note centripetal distribution of rash

Day 3 of rash

Lesions are in different stages of development

Healthy adult with varicella

Healthy adult with varicella

Pregnant woman with varicella

Figure 6-15 Chickenpox presentation.
Courtesy of the Centers for Disease Control and Prevention

prehospital care practitioners must wear PPE appropriate for contact and aerosol precautions. This includes an N95 mask, eye protection, goggles, and gown. Ideally, persons managing patients with smallpox will have been immunized.

The smallpox vaccination program in the United States was stopped in 1972. The residual immunity provided by this vaccination program is unknown, and it is suggested that individuals whose last immunization was 40 years ago will likely now be susceptible to contracting smallpox. In case of a public health emergency, the United States has stockpiles of vaccines that can be released for mass immunization of the public. Vaccination within 4 days of exposure has been shown to offer some

protection against contracting the illness and substantial protection against a fatal outcome.

In the prehospital setting, the patient with smallpox is managed with supportive care. The recommended PPE must be worn at all times, and it is imperative that there is no breach in infection control procedures. Hospitals with the appropriate isolation facilities and properly trained staff should be identified in the community. The receiving facility must be contacted to inform the staff of the intention to transport the confirmed or suspected case of smallpox to their facility so that proper precautions can be taken to prevent virus transmission. Identifying a patient with smallpox would be considered a public health emergency of enormous significance.

Proper removal of PPE without a breach in infection control procedures is important for the safety of the prehospital care practitioner. All contaminated disposable medical waste must be properly bagged, labeled, and disposed of as other regulated medical waste. Reusable medical equipment must be cleaned after use according to standard protocol, either by autoclaving or by subjecting the equipment to high-level disinfection. Environmental surfaces need to be cleaned by an approved EPA-registered detergent disinfectant. Air decontamination or fumigation of the emergency vehicle is not required.

Ebola Virus

Ebola virus causes Ebola virus disease (EVD), a type of **viral hemorrhagic fever**, similar to the Lassa, dengue, yellow, and Marburg fevers. This is a deadly disease with outbreaks occurring most commonly in Africa. The virus is transmitted by contact with infected bats and nonhuman primates. It initially spreads when humans come into contact with the blood, body fluids, or tissues of an infected animal. It then spreads from person to person through direct contact with blood or body fluids via broken skin or mucous membranes (e.g., eyes, nose, mouth). The Ebola virus gained worldwide attention in 2014 when an EVD outbreak spread throughout West Africa, causing over 11,000 deaths among over 28,000 reported cases between 2013 and 2016, including several in the United States and other Western countries.

Clinically, EVD initially manifests after a 2- to 21-day incubation period with fevers, chills, generalized malaise, and muscle aches and then progresses to GI symptoms, including abdominal pain, vomiting, and diarrhea; neurologic symptoms, including headache and confusion; and respiratory symptoms, including cough, chest pain, and shortness of breath. In severe cases, hemorrhagic symptoms and generalized coagulopathy at the peak of illness may develop. Death occurs from multiorgan failure, sepsis, electrolyte abnormalities, and hypovolemic shock, primarily from GI volume loss. Although the case fatality rate varies significantly among strains and different outbreaks, the 2013–2016 West African outbreak had a final case fatality rate of below 40%, versus around 75% at the outbreak's start and over 90% in some prior outbreaks. This rate was suspected to have improved due to improvements in caring for patients with EVD, primarily aggressive replacement of GI volume and electrolyte losses.

Transport of patients suspected to have EVD poses a significant risk to EMS personnel due to the highly infectious nature of the virus. Body fluids from symptomatic patients contain extremely large amounts of active virus, and only a small exposure is needed to infect an individual. A review of the West African outbreak showed that 3.9% of cases were among health care workers who became infected while caring for EVD patients.

The CDC has published specific guidelines on PPE use for transporting EVD patients. The CDC recommends skin protection with multiple layers (disposable scrubs, impermeable gown, over-apron, multiple layers of gloves, and boot covers) and respiratory/mucous membrane protection, with a **powered air-purifying respirator (PAPR)** and hood preferred over N95 mask and eye protection, analogous to level C PPE. These recommendations may be updated if another outbreak occurs. Extensive training on EVD PPE and direct supervision of donning/doffing procedures by experienced observers are strongly recommended.

EMS agencies affiliated with special pathogens hospitals had developed equipment and plans for transporting critically ill patients with highly contagious diseases before the 2013–2016 EVD outbreak. Afterward, they published reports on their experiences treating and transporting actual and suspected EVD patients. These reports made many specific and helpful recommendations for transporting EVD patients.

Based on experience gained in the 2013–2016 outbreak, medical management of EVD patients now focuses primarily on symptom control and oral repletion of GI fluids and electrolyte losses. New therapies, including antiviral and immunomodulatory medications and vaccines, may improve survival rates, but their efficacy is still under investigation. Advances in supportive care interventions, such as IV fluids; lab monitoring of electrolytes, cell counts, and viral levels; antibiotics; and intubation/ventilation, may also be helpful. However, these measures significantly increase the risk of infection to health care practitioners. Isolation rooms should be used for contaminated patients.

An Ebola vaccine is available for adults but is limited to health care personnel.

EMS Management of EVD

- Use appropriate PPE (with strict attention paid to donning/doffing procedure and recommendation for a PAPR rather than a negative-pressure mask for better practitioner protection and comfort during long transports).
- Minimize the number of personnel providing direct patient care.
- Isolate the driver compartment of the ambulance from the patient compartment with an improvised positive-pressure system.
- Cover all equipment and surfaces within the patient compartment of the ambulance with thick plastic sheets to limit contamination.
- Further isolate patients within a contamination-limiting suit or capsule.
- Carefully decontaminate the ambulance and equipment afterward by using disinfectant wipes (as opposed to spraying down surfaces with pressurized water, which could aerosolize virus particles).

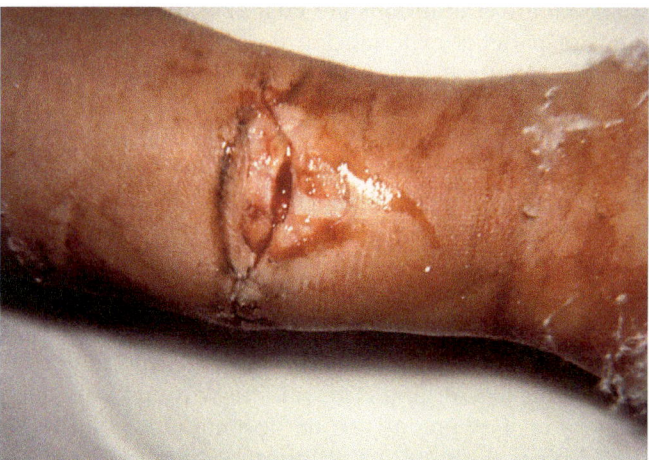

Figure 6-16 Volar view of a patient's right arm, which had sustained a penetrating wound due to a compound fracture, and though treated, developed what is known as wound botulism.
Courtesy of the Centers for Disease Control and Prevention

Botulinum Toxin

C. botulinum, the bacterial agent that causes botulism, produces a neurotoxin that causes paralysis. Types of exposures include ingestion of contaminated food and contamination of wounds with the bacterium (**Figure 6-16**). All forms are considered medical emergencies and can be lethal. In the case of bioterrorism, infiltration of food sources or the water supply can cause many people to become sick. Even small amounts of the bacteria can devastate large populated areas.

Care for the patient with botulism is supportive, with the administration of antitoxin in the hospital. Early use of antitoxin will minimize further deterioration but cannot reverse existing paralysis. Hospitals may not have antitoxin immediately available, so local protocols must include a process for obtaining the appropriate therapies. The antitoxin is available from the CDC.

A patient with botulism usually has nausea, blurred vision, fatigue, slurred speech, muscle weakness, and paralysis. Symptoms can occur within hours or several days after exposure. Report any increase in patients with similar complaints to the appropriate receiving facilities and agencies.

Prehospital care practitioners caring for victims of botulism would need to be vigilant about airway compromise and insufficient ventilation. Patients may be unable to manage their secretions or maintain a patent airway. Because of diaphragm paralysis, patients may not be able to generate an adequate tidal volume; thus, a rise in end-tidal carbon dioxide levels may be an early sign that the patient's ventilatory effort is compromised. Respiratory difficulty may be exacerbated by having the patient supine or in semirecumbent position. Patients experiencing respiratory difficulty should be intubated and adequately ventilated.

Standard precautions are adequate for the management of patients experiencing the effects of botulinum toxicity because it is not a contagious disease. Botulism aerosols degrade readily in the environment, and it is anticipated that after delivery in a terrorist incident, substantial inactivation will occur after 2 days. Responders to an overt aerosol dissemination event would require level A PPE suitable for a hazardous environment if working in a hot zone or warm zone.

Because the aerosol can persist for approximately 2 days under average weather conditions, victims who have been exposed to botulinum aerosol require decontamination by clothing removal and washing with soap and water. Equipment can be decontaminated using a 0.1% hypochlorite bleach solution. Patients will not require isolation after arrival at the hospital, but critical care services may be needed for patients requiring mechanical ventilation.

Pandemic Preparedness and Response: Crisis Standards of Care

Large-scale biologic disasters, including pandemics, will likely deplete a region's scarce resources, such as ventilators, ICU beds, specialized personnel, and technical resources. Such situations may require adjustment to routine practices to help limit death and suffering.

Standards of care fall along three levels. According to the Association of American Medical Colleges, these are conventional, contingency, and crisis standards of care. Conventional care, or everyday care, is the norm. Contingency care involves adjustments to everyday care, but the level of care for an individual patient remains functionally equivalent. Crisis standards of care are applied when a disaster results in sustained resource shortages that are severe enough to require a change in how health care is delivered across a region, putting the practitioner or patient at risk of a poor outcome.

Crisis standards of care must incorporate the complex balance of the need for resources, the ability to deliver health care, and public health and be strongly grounded in ethics. As outlined in a 2020 National Academies of Science, Engineering, and Medicine report, crisis standards of care seek to "[extend] the availability of key resources and [minimize] the impact of shortages on clinical care." Much like disaster triage, it is understood that by striving to save as many lives as possible some individual patients will die who would have otherwise survived. Therefore, experts emphasize that a key preparedness goal is never to need crisis standards of care.

Resource Shortages That Could Lead to Crisis Conditions

- Supplies, such as medications, N95 masks, dialysis equipment, ventilators, beds, and cardiac monitors
- Staff, particularly those with specialized training (e.g., critical care)
- Space, which may be a shortfall if there are too many patients for local hospitals to accommodate

It is important to monitor supply shortages and conserve resources before they run out.

How Can Resource Shortfalls Be Addressed?

- Adaptation of practices
- Rationing decisions
- Substitution of similar supplies
- Conservation of existing resources (e.g., smaller doses, restrictions on use)
- Adaptation of one resource for another purpose
- Reuse of resources
- Reallocation of a resource from a patient with a poor prognosis to one with a better prognosis

CASE STUDY

Case Overview

You are working on an advanced life support (ALS) transport unit when dispatched to the international headquarters of a well-known media company for a sick person in the health suite. Dispatch advises they are adding two additional reports of several ill people with fever and respiratory symptoms. This case study will focus on response to a potential biologic emergency, including EMS practitioner safety considerations.

What are your initial concerns based on the dispatch information?

The initial impression begins when the dispatch information is received. EMS practitioner safety concerns include the following:
PPE considerations

- Potential infectious agents and transmission routes
- Precautions to minimize the risk of exposure
- Importance of decontamination procedures (for recent exposures)

Initial Information

Upon arrival, you are met by the occupational health director. Five people presented this morning with fevers and shortness of breath. All the patients work in the accounts receivable department. A suspicious package was received yesterday. The substance was sent to a lab by law enforcement, and the results are still pending. The pathogen is unknown. You are led into the health room, where you find five adults in varying degrees of respiratory distress, from mild to moderate.

What are your initial concerns?

- PPE
- Available resources
- Any obstacles
- Triage
- Contact precautions
- Transport decisions

What are the PPE requirements when handling patients with unknown respiratory illness?

- PPE should include respiratory protection (at least an N95 respirator), full face protection, a gown, and gloves.

- The potential use of level C suits (or fluid-impermeable gowns) and proper donning and doffing will be important to reduce practitioner infection.
- You should be open to changing the PPE level as the situation evolves.

When should you don the PPE?

- EMS personnel should don all PPE before entering the facility to avoid contamination from anyone who has contacted the patients.

What source control measures should you consider in this environment?

- Droplet masks on patients
- Bag-valve mask and CPAP masks with filters

What would happen if you transported a patient to a closer, minor-care clinic versus a trauma hospital?

- Transporting an infectious disease patient to an alternative facility, such as an urgent care clinic, could put more people at risk.

What modifications should be made to the ambulance patient compartment?

The ambulance patient compartment's exhaust fan should be on a high setting; if possible, the driver's compartment should be isolated and the fan set to high, with the recirculation mode off.

Given the unknown pathogen in this case and the critically ill respiratory patients, it is reasonable to drape the patient compartment. The U.S. Department of Health and Human Services recommends draping the patient compartment specifically for suspected smallpox, novel influenza, Ebola virus, and other viral hemorrhagic fevers.

In theory, the ambulance should be isolated and draped, if possible. However, this process takes a lot of time, and it might be more expeditious to decontaminate the ambulance after patient transport.

On-Scene Actions

Upon arrival, you are the first unit on the scene. One practitioner will be incident command, and the other will serve as the triage officer. You complete the LCAN report.

Location

- Health room in the international headquarters of a media company

Conditions

- Clinic personnel state that five patients arrived within the past 2 hours with cough and shortness of breath, and now one is vomiting blood.
- The five patients are visibly anxious and upset.

Actions

- Establish command and begin triage. Use your regional triage system.

Needs

- Identify reinforcement needs.
- Additional ambulances are needed to transport patients. Once the exact number of patients is known, specialty transport units should be called in as soon as possible.
- What alternate transport methods could be used? Air medical could be an option with the appropriate PPE.

What additional precautions or concerns may be warranted based on initial observations?

- Scene safety is critical, and EMS practitioners, first responders, patients, and bystanders should be protected from exposure when working on an emergency scene.
- Securing the area is critical to limit exposure.
- As these individuals may have been exposed to an unknown substance, law enforcement should also be requested.

What equipment do you need?

- As the first ambulance on scene, what equipment would be reasonable to treat patients with infectious diseases?
- How much additional equipment could be carried in with the EMS team (e.g., PPE, blankets, oxygen, and airway treatment supplies)?
- How would you approach the patients and inform them of the need to wear appropriate PPE?

Initial Assessment

While waiting for the additional ALS ambulances to arrive, you and your partner began triaging the five patients:

- Patient 1 is now unresponsive and requires ventilation with a bag-valve mask.
- Patient 2 requires noninvasive ventilation.
- Patient 3 is on a nonrebreather with oxygen saturation levels in the low 90s.
- Patient 4 is vomiting bloody material.
- Patient 5 reports subjective shortness of breath and is not hypoxic.

What triage considerations pertain to the current situation?

- Importance of a rapid and accurate assessment of patients
- Triage categories and criteria
- Establishment of an initial patient count (if known) to determine the number and kind of additional resources needed
- Special considerations for a biologic emergency such as higher-level PPE and any contaminated materials (e.g., body fluids)

What should you consider with regard to additional resources?

- Is an EMS supervisor/physician needed?
- Notify receiving facilities.
- Attempt to obtain additional information about the contents of the envelope.
- Will you need to request additional resources? In this case, five patients need transport. You are already there with one ambulance; two additional ambulances have also arrived; therefore, two additional units should be requested to expedite the response.
- How would you manage the scene in a rural setting without specialized units? Having the appropriate PPE is critical to the safety of all responders. EMS personnel who do not have the appropriate equipment could contact local medical clinics or the nearest hospital for appropriate PPE.

How do scene assessment and awareness apply to this case?

Remember, attending to detail and utilizing a team approach to EMS practitioner safety when responding to infectious diseases or biologic disasters is extremely important.

Patient Triage Review

How many (more) patients do you expect?

- Number of patients: five
- However, more patients could have encountered the 5 patients in the health suite (5 patients could easily turn into 10 or 50).
- You know you have at least five patients at various triage levels (green, yellow, red).

What triage categories and life threats do you observe during the patient primary surveys?

- Triage may be challenging and will be performed as patients are accessed.
- Patients 1 and 4 are the highest priority patients and should be transported emergently.
- Patients 2, 3, and 5, although in need of prehospital management, can be considered lower priority patients.

How would raising the criticality of the patients affect the patients' treatment?

If an adult and a pediatric patient were both critical (red) and requiring ventilatory support during transport, how would the PPE change?

- HEPA (or bacterial/viral) filter on ventilator circuits, endotracheal (ET) tubes, CPAP/BPAP masks, or bag-valve masks

Patient Transport

What complications may occur during transport?

Many complications could make traditional medical evacuation difficult, impossible, or unrealistic. EMS practitioners may become contaminated. EMS personnel must identify the considerations when planning to move or receive patients to ensure the safe handling of all involved and avoid further contamination. You must recognize all available options and understand the three key elements of planned and impromptu evacuation:

1. Appreciating the current condition
2. Maintaining awareness of all the available resources and their capabilities
3. Knowing the desired end goal and communicating effectively

What about communications in this environment?

Hands-free radios or cell phones should be used *and* decontaminated after each transport.

Is air medical transport appropriate for these patients?

This is dependent on the transport times and available PPE resources.

How many patients can you safely transport in your ambulance?

- This may depend on organizational and state guidelines for transporting multiple patients in an ambulance during this disaster.
- From a safety standpoint, it would be more prudent to transport each patient individually. Although in a resource-limited setting, this may not be possible.

Transport Destination

Where would the patients be transported to and why?

- The patients should be transported to a health care facility capable of managing infectious diseases.

What would happen if you transported a patient to a closer, minor-care clinic versus a trauma hospital?

- Transporting an infectious disease patient to an alternative facility, such as an urgent care clinic, could put more people at risk.

CASE WRAP UP

In total, five patients were transported to a hospital capable of managing communicable diseases. The patients were evaluated and treated for inhalational anthrax. Unfortunately, two did not survive.

The public health department was notified of the infectious disease per organizational policies and procedures. Law enforcement was also notified, given the report of recent exposure to the unknown white powder.

After the incident, you and your team decontaminated yourselves and the ambulance. The following safety measures were performed:

- Sanitizing wipes were used for the rapid sanitization of practitioners, equipment, stretcher, and ambulance. This was followed with aerosolizing sanitizers.
- At all stages of the decontamination process, the practitioners were monitored for signs of fatigue or errors by a dedicated safety officer/team.
- Once all practitioners, equipment, and the unit were decontaminated, all materials were bagged, labeled, and properly disposed of at the receiving hospital.
- All practitioners were enrolled in a monitoring program with their safety officer in which daily screenings of temperature and disease signs/symptoms were monitored and reported.
- If any signs or symptoms were to develop, the practitioner would be isolated/quarantined and the appropriate public health entity notified.

SUMMARY

- Proper PPE selection, donning, and doffing are key to responding to an infectious disease outbreak or a biologic disaster.
- Strict adherence to decontamination guidelines is paramount when responding to an infectious disease outbreak or a biologic disaster.
- Transmission-based precautions used to minimize the risk of exposure to infectious agents include contact precautions, droplet precautions, and aerosol precautions.
- Ambulance modification may be required when transporting highly infectious patients.
- Donning and doffing PPE is done to ensure the user is adequately protected.
- Level A PPE offers the highest level of respiratory and skin protection. Responding in level A PPE for a prolonged period is unreasonable, regardless of the threat.
- Decontamination strategies that can be used based on the specific situation include decontamination of clothing by washing with soap and water; decontamination of equipment using a 0.1% hypochlorite bleach solution; autoclaving or high-level disinfection of reusable medical equipment; careful decontamination of ambulance and equipment with disinfectant wipes, ultraviolet radiation, or disinfectant misting (dry fogging); and cleaning of environmental surfaces with EPA-registered detergent/disinfectant.
- Ambulance modification may be necessary when transporting highly infectious patients, as in the case of wet Ebola.
- Bioterrorism is when biologic agents are used on humans, animals, and crops to cause fear and harm.
- Bioterrorism agents can be dispersed through various means, including aerosolized agents (most likely), contaminated food or water supply, letters or packages, infected animals used as a vector, and human-to-human contact.
- The CDC categorizes bioterrorism agents by priority level, based on their impact. Category A bioterrorism agents pose the highest risk to national security and public health and have been weaponized by countries/terrorist organizations.
- Emergency responders can experience bioterrorism in two ways: (1) overt release of a biohazard agent and (2) response to a victim of a bioterrorist event.
- Biologic triage for highly infectious pathogens aims to help control transmission, minimize the spread of illness, and assist with resource allocation and prioritization. Biologic triage categories include susceptible but not exposed, exposed but not yet infectious, infectious, removed by death or recovery, and protected by vaccination or prophylactic medication.
- According to the Association of American Medical Colleges, standards of care fall along three levels: conventional care, contingency care, and crisis standards of care.
- Crisis standards of care are applied when a disaster or epidemic results in sustained resource shortages that are severe enough to require a change in how health care is delivered across a region that puts the practitioner or patient at risk of a poor outcome.
- Resource shortfalls can be managed through adaptation of practices, rationing decisions, substitution of similar supplies, conservation of existing resources (e.g., smaller doses, restrictions on use), adaptation of one resource for another purpose, reuse of resources, and reallocation of a resource from a patient with a poor prognosis to one with a better prognosis.

References and Additional Resources

Arnon SS, Schechter R, Inglesby TV, et al. Botulinum toxin as a biological weapon: medical and public health management. *JAMA*. 2001;285:1059–1070.

ASPR TRACIE. *Crisis Standard of Care Brief: Healthcare Providers*. April 2022. https://files.asprtracie.hhs.gov/documents/aspr-tracie-csc-brief-healthcare-providers.pdf. Accessed April 18, 2023.

Basler CF. Molecular pathogenesis of viral hemorrhagic fever. *Semin Immunopathol*. 2017;39(5):551–561.

Cenciarelli O, Gabbarini V, Pietropaoli S, et al. Viral bioterrorism: learning the lesson of Ebola virus in West Africa 2013–2015. *Virus Res*. 2015;210:318–326.

Centers for Disease Control and Prevention. Bioterrorism agents/diseases. https://emergency.cdc.gov/agent/agentlist-category.asp. Accessed May 9, 2023.

Centers for Disease Control and Prevention. How to safely remove personal protective equipment (PPE). https://www.cdc.gov/hai/pdfs/ppe/PPE-Sequence.pdf. Accessed May 9, 2023.

Centers for Disease Control and Prevention. Sequence for putting on personal protective equipment (PPE). https://www.cdc.gov/hai/pdfs/ppe/PPE-Sequence.pdf. Accessed May 9, 2023.

Centers for Disease Control and Prevention. *Smallpox Response Plan and Guidelines*. Version 3.0, Guide C, Part 1. Centers for Disease Control and Prevention; 2008:1–13.

Centers for Disease Control and Prevention. *Smallpox Response Plan and Guidelines*. Version 3.0, Guide F. Centers for Disease Control and Prevention; 2003:1–10.

Centers for Disease Control and Prevention, National Center for Emerging and Zoonotic Infectious Diseases, Division of Healthcare Quality Promotion. Guidance on personal protective equipment (PPE) to be used by healthcare workers during management of patients with confirmed Ebola or persons under investigation (PUIs) for Ebola who are clinically unstable or have bleeding, vomiting, or diarrhea in U.S. hospitals, including procedures for donning and doffing PPE. Reviewed August 30, 2018. https://www.cdc.gov/vhf/ebola/healthcare-us/ppe/guidance.html. Accessed July 19, 2023.

Coltart CE, Lindsey B, Ghinai I, Johnson AM, Heymann DL. The Ebola outbreak, 2013–2016: old lessons for new epidemics. *Philos Trans R Soc Lond B Biol Sci*. 2017;372(1721):20160297.

Duraffour S, Malvy D, Sissoko D. How to treat Ebola virus infections? A lesson from the field. *Curr Opin Virol*. 2017;24:9–15.

Feldmann H, Geisbert TW. Ebola haemorrhagic fever. *Lancet*. 2011;377:849–862.

Franz DR, Jahrling PB, Friedlander AM, et al. Clinical recognition and management of patients exposed to biological warfare agents. *JAMA*. 1997;278(5):399–411.

Henderson DA, Inglesby TV, Bartlett JG. Smallpox as a biological weapon: medical and public health management. *JAMA*. 1999;281(22):2127–2137.

Hick JL, Hanfling D, Burstein JL, Markham J, Macintyre AG, Barbera JA. Protective equipment for health care facility decontamination personnel: regulations, risks, and recommendations. *Ann Emerg Med*. 2003;42(3):370–380.

Inglesby TV, Dennis DT, Henderson DA. Plague as a biological weapon: medical and public health management. *JAMA*. 2000;283(17):2281–2290.

Inglesby TV, O'Toole T, Henderson DA, et al. Anthrax as a biological weapon, 2002: updated recommendations for management. *JAMA*. 2002;287:2236–2252.

Isakov A, Miles W, Gibbs S, Lowe J, Jamison A, Swansiger R. Transport and management of patients with confirmed or suspected Ebola virus disease. *Ann Emerg Med*. 2015;66(3):297–305.

Keim M, Kaufmann AF. Principles for emergency response to bioterrorism. *Ann Emerg Med*. 1999;34(2):177–182.

Kman NE, Nelson RN. Infectious agents of bioterrorism: a review for emergency physicians. *Emerg Med Clin North Am*. 2008;26:517–547.

Lowe JJ, Jelden KC, Schenarts PJ, et al. Considerations for safe EMS transport of patients infected with Ebola virus. *Prehosp Emerg Care*. 2015;19(2):179–183.

National Academies of Sciences, Engineering, and Medicine. *Rapid Expert Consultation on Crisis Standards of Care for the COVID-19 Pandemic*. The National Academies Press; March 28, 2020.

National Association of Emergency Medical Technicians. *Prehospital Trauma Life Support*. 10th ed. Jones & Bartlett Learning; 2023.

Stern EJ, Uhde KB, Shadomy SV, Messonnier N. Conference report on public health and clinical guidelines for anthrax. *Emerging Infect Dis*. 2008;14(4).

World Health Organization. *Health Aspects of Chemical and Biological Weapons*. World Health Organization; 1970.

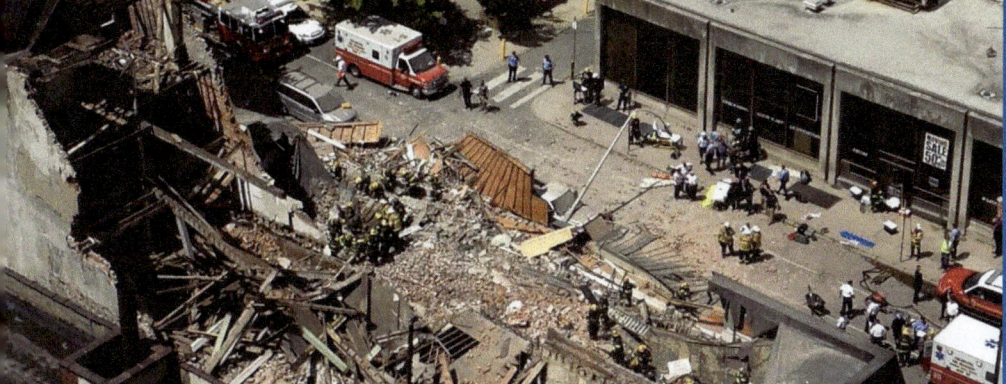

Chemical and Radiologic/ Nuclear Disasters

LESSON OBJECTIVES

At the completion of this lesson, you should be able to do the following:

· Identify the scenarios in which secondary contamination with a chemical agent can occur.

· Describe the decontamination principles in chemical and radiologic/nuclear disasters.

· List the management steps in chemical and radiologic/nuclear disasters.

What Are Hazardous Materials?

A **hazardous material (hazmat)** is any substance that poses an unreasonable threat to health, safety, or the environment. Hazardous materials include corrosives, radioactive matter, and flammable materials, and they can be inhaled, ingested, or absorbed through the skin. Exposure to hazardous materials poses a threat to all communities. These materials are found, for example, in local refineries, factories, and industrial plants that produce various chemicals. These dangerous goods pass along our highways, railways, and airports as they travel long distances. Hazardous materials are also manufactured illicitly in neighborhoods and rural meth labs. EMS practitioners must maintain a keen awareness of these threats when approaching a perilous scene or situation or when a patient's cardinal presentation indicates there may have been exposure to a hazardous material.

Similarities Between Management of Hazmat Disasters

Chemical and radiologic/nuclear disaster management share many similarities, including the concepts of scene safety, zones of control, personal protective equipment (PPE), and decontamination.

Hazmat Incident Identification

The occurrence of a hazmat incident can be initially difficult to identify. Dispatch information regarding the number of patients and any similarities in their signs and symptoms can indicate the need for immediate identification of appropriate safety precautions and additional resources.

At the scene, low-lying clouds, smoke, unusual fog patterns, odors, or air density should heighten suspicion that a hazmat incident may have occurred. Multiple patients with similar presenting signs and symptoms, including significant skin or eye irritation, respiratory difficulties, and seizures, indicate a potential hazmat incident and should serve as triggers of a possible hazmat scene and prompt EMS practitioners to initiate special precautions.

Time of Dispatch

At the time of dispatch and while en route to the scene of a hazmat incident, EMS practitioners should begin assessing information and taking stock of their resources:

- Note the weather conditions and wind direction.
- Gauge the proximity of highly populated areas relative to the exposure area.
- Determine the number, location, and abilities of receiving facilities.
- Review the type of hazardous material and the amount to which victims are thought to have been exposed.
- Estimate the number of people who have been exposed or are at risk of exposure.

Approaching the Hazmat Scene

If possible, approach the scene from an uphill, upwind direction if hazardous materials are suspected. Limit access to the scene to prevent exposure. Request assistance from appropriate additional resources before accessing the scene. Use available technologies (e.g., traffic cameras, binoculars) to remotely assess for evidence of hazards. Use the "thumb rule": If you hold up your thumb and can see the incident or hazard around it, you are too close. This practice allows you to avoid contamination of responding resources. It is important to identify the source of the hazard and the conditions surrounding the incident, such as the integrity of any packages or containers or **chemical placards** on vehicles, packages, and containers. Once you recognize that an area or patient may have been subject to hazmat exposure, immediately don PPE and notify the appropriate agencies, make resource requests, and initiate the incident command system (ICS) as appropriate.

Chemical Placards

In the United States, the Department of Transportation (DOT) regulates the transportation of hazardous materials, including labeling such materials during transport. The agency sets the standards that specify the types of containers for various kinds of hazardous materials and their modes of transport, labeling, and accompanying documentation. The presence of a hazardous material is identified by placards, shipping papers, labels, or pictographs that specify the type of hazardous agent present, the nature and degree of the medical compromise expected if exposure occurs, and the signs and symptoms of exposure.

A placard is a diamond-shaped sign affixed to a transport vehicle (**Figure 7-1**). The placard is color coded to identify the hazardous agent as flammable, combustible, poisonous, radioactive, gaseous, explosive, oxidizing, infectious, or corrosive (**Table 7-1**). Each placard carries a

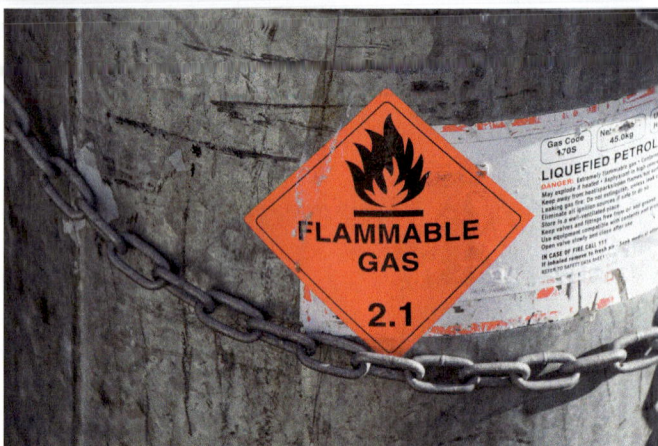

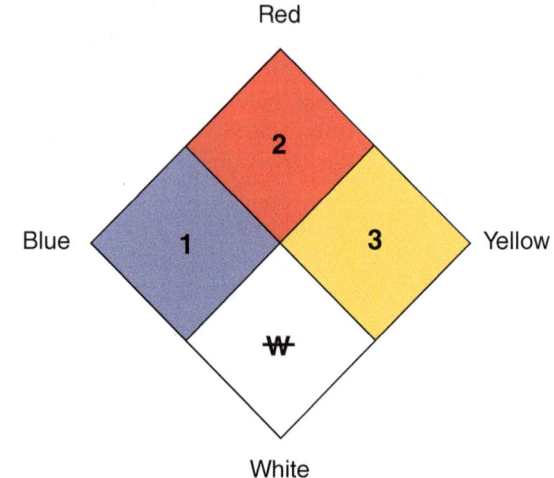

Figure 7-1 Chemical placards on vehicles, packages, and containers offer information about the substances that may be involved in the incident.

Table 7-1 Classes of Hazardous Materials

Class/Division	Notes
Class 1: Explosives Division 1.1: Mass detonation hazard Division 1.2: Mass detonation hazard with fragments Division 1.3: Fire hazard with minor blast or projectile hazard Division 1.4: Explosive substances that present no significant hazard Division 1.5: Very insensitive explosives Division 1.6: Extremely insensitive explosives	Explosive placards and labels are orange and have a symbol showing an exploding ball with fragments on the top and a division number (1.1 to 1.6) on the bottom. The word *explosive* or a four-digit ID number appears in the center of the symbol.
Class 2: Gases Division 2.1: Flammable gases Division 2.2: Nonflammable gases Division 2.3: Poisonous gases	Compressed or liquefied gas placards and labels are red (flammable), green (nonflammable), or white (poison); have a fire symbol, gas cylinder symbol, or skull and crossbones on the top; and have a division number (2.1 to 2.3) on the bottom. These symbols have *flammable gas*, *nonflammable gas*, or *poison gas* labeling or a four-digit ID number in the center.
Class 3: Flammable or combustible liquids Division 3.1: Liquids with flash points <0°F Division 3.2: Liquids with flash points from 0°F to 73°F Division 3.3: Liquids with flash points from 73°F to 141°F Combustible liquids	Flammable or combustible liquids placards and labels are red, have a flame symbol on the top, and a division number (3.1 to 3.3) on the bottom. They have the wording *flammable liquid* or *combustible liquid* or a four-digit ID number in the center.
Class 4: Flammable solids Division 4.1: Flammable solids Division 4.2: Spontaneously combustible or pyrophoric solids and liquids Division 4.3: Dangerous when wet	Flammable solid placards and labels are red-and-white striped (flammable solids), red over white (spontaneously combustible solids and liquids), or blue (dangerous when wet); have a flame symbol on the top; and have a division number (4.1 to 4.3) on the bottom. They have the wording *flammable solid*, *spontaneously combustible*, or *dangerous when wet* or a four-digit ID number in the center.
Class 5: Oxidizing substances Division 5.1: Oxidizers Division 5.2: Organic peroxides	Oxidizing substances placards and labels are yellow, have a symbol showing an O with flames on the top, and a division number (5.1 to 5.2) on the bottom. They have the wording *oxidizer* or *organic peroxide* or a four-digit ID number in the center.
Class 6: Poisonous and infectious substances Division 6.1: Poisons Division 6.2: Infectious substances	Poison liquid and solid material and infectious material placards and labels are white; have either skull and crossbones, biomedical symbol, or grain stock with an *X* through it (depending on material) on the top; and a division number (6.1 to 6.2) on the bottom. These symbols have the wording *poison*, *infectious material*, *keep away from foodstuffs* or a four-digit ID number in the center.

(continues)

Table 7-1 Classes of Hazardous Materials (*continued*)

Class/Division	Notes
Class 7: Radioactive substances	Radioactive materials placards and labels are yellow over white, have the radioactive propeller symbol on the top, and the number 7 on the bottom. Labels must identify the radionuclide and the amount of activity in the package. They will have the Roman numerals I, II, or III in the center to identify the level of hazard and type of container and space to write in specific information. The I, II, or III numbering designates the amount of radiation detectable from outside the package. Labels have the wording *radioactive material* or a four-digit ID number in the center.
Class 8: Corrosive materials	Corrosive materials placards and labels are white over black, have a symbol showing a test tube spilling liquid onto a human thumb, and a piece of steel on the top and have the number 8 on the bottom. The word *corrosive* or a four-digit ID number appears in the center.
Class 9: Miscellaneous hazardous materials	Miscellaneous hazardous materials placards and labels are black-and-white striped over white and have the number 9 on the bottom. They have a four-digit ID number in the center.

four-digit identification number that allows the agent to be identified quickly when cross-referenced against print and online reference sources such as the DOT's *Emergency Response Guidebook* (*ERG*). The Occupational Safety and Health Administration (OSHA) requires chemical manufacturers to create **material safety data sheets (MSDS)** for every chemical developed, stored, and used in the United States. These MSDS forms provide instructions for the safe handling and storage of the chemical and outline emergency actions to take if an exposure occurs. These sheets must always remain with the chemical.

All health care clinicians must be able to interpret hazmat labeling or have immediate access to guides or agencies to assist in identification. Clinicians who cannot recognize hazardous product labeling risk unintentionally becoming contaminated themselves. The Centers for Disease Control and Prevention's Agency for Toxic Substances and Disease Registry maintains an online set of resources for emergency responders in the United States (https://www.atsdr.cdc.gov/emergencyresponse/index.html).

Regulatory Agency Notification

It is important to notify receiving facilities and local, state, and national agencies of hazardous materials and possible weapons of mass destruction (WMDs) as soon as you recognize them. Agencies such as OSHA and the Environmental Protection Agency (EPA) develop and mandate personnel training and local, state, and federal emergency plans. An OSHA regulation known as the Standard on Hazardous Waste Operations and Emergency Response (HAZWOPER) provides guidelines for developing and complying with safety protocols and procedures regarding the cleanup of hazardous materials for governmental and nongovernmental personnel who make, store, or dispose of hazardous materials, or are first responders to hazmat incidents. The National Fire Protection Association (NFPA) also identifies standards for safety competency related to scene management for first responders.

Zones of Operation

Proximity to the threat is often described in terms of zones of operations: the hot zone, the warm zone, and the cold zone (**Figure 7-2**).

In a chemical, radiologic, or nuclear disaster, the hot (red) zone is the environment contaminated with hazardous gas, vapor, aerosol, liquid, powder, or radiation level of more than 2 milliroentgens per hour (mR/h). Level A PPE is most often used in the hot zone.

The warm (yellow) zone is the area where the concentration of the offending agent is limited or the radiation level is 2 mR/h. EMS practitioners are still at heightened risk for exposure if working in this area, as the agent is carried from the hot zone on victims, other practitioners, and equipment.

The cold (green) zone is the area that is not contaminated (or with radiation < 2 mR/h). In this area, there is no risk of exposure and thus no specific level of PPE is required beyond standard precautions.

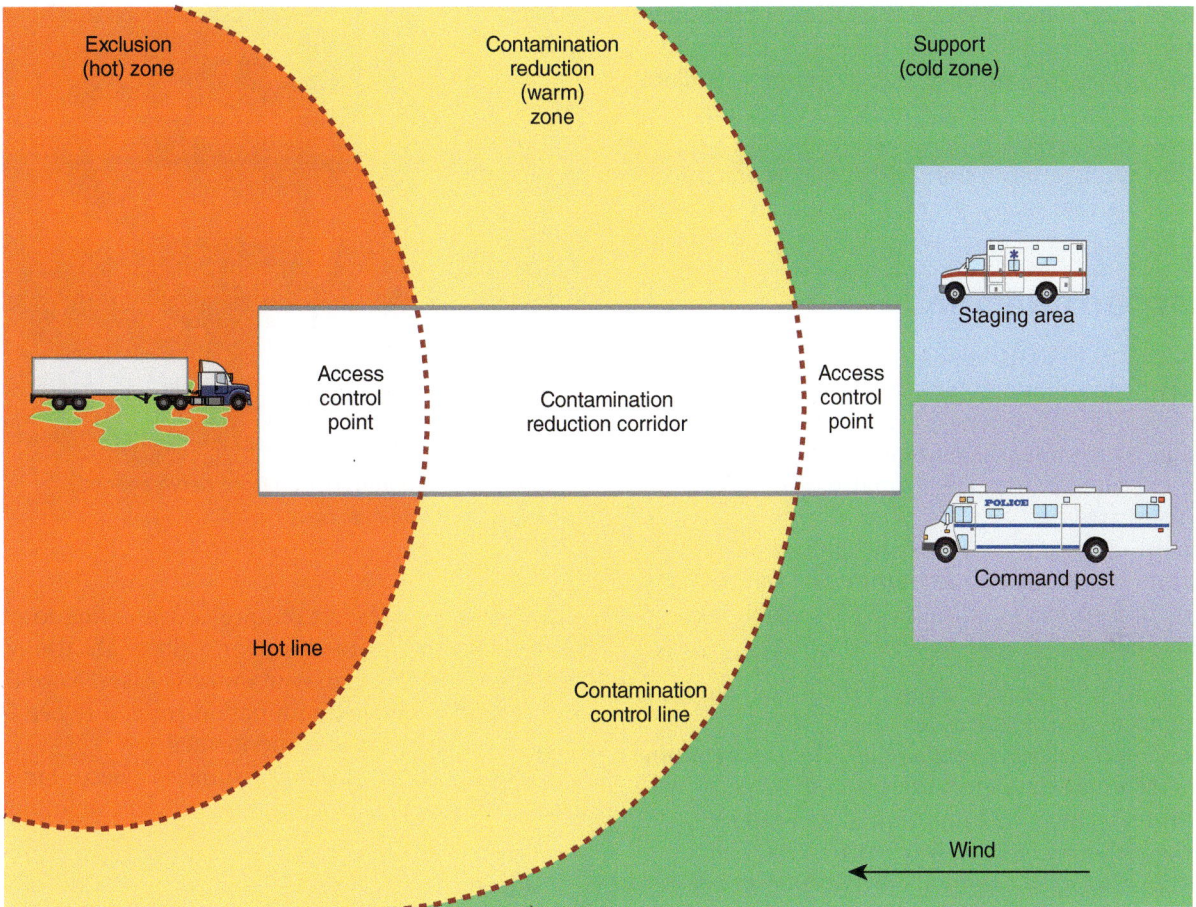

Figure 7-2 The scene of a WMD or hazmat incident is generally divided into hot, warm, and cold zones. The command post and staging area should both be located within the cold zone.

© National Association of Emergency Medical Technicians (NAEMT)

Personal Protective Equipment (PPE)

PPE is selected based on the threat of exposure to the chemical agent (see Table 6-1). Level A PPE is appropriate for EMS practitioners entering the hot zone until the specific agents in use and their concentrations are known. Once the agent has been identified, incident command may decide to move to lower levels of PPE (B or C), particularly for practitioners tasked with carrying out decontamination or working in the warm zone.

The PPE available for use in chemical hazards will offer some protection from radioactive particulate contamination but no protection from high-energy radiation sources (e.g., damaged reactor, nuclear blast at ground zero). If radioactive gases are present, a self-contained breathing apparatus (SCBA) will offer the highest protection (**Table 7-2**). If aerosols are present, an **air-purifying respirator (APR)** may be adequate to prevent internal contamination. An N95 mask will offer some protection

Table 7-2 PPE in Radiologic/Nuclear Disaster

PPE Item	Protects Against
SCBA	Radioactive gases
APR	Aerosols
N95 mask	Inhaled particulates
Standard splash-resistant suit	Particulates that emit alpha radiation, some protection from beta radiation

© National Association of Emergency Medical Technicians (NAEMT)

from inhaled particulates. A standard splash-resistant suit will protect against particulates that emit alpha radiation and offer some protection from beta radiation; however, it does not offer protection from gamma radiation or neutrons.

None of the typical PPE protects from a high-energy point source of radiation. New materials that may offer some protection from low-level gamma radiation for EMS-practitioner PPE are under investigation. It is important to remember that agency-specific protocols should always determine the zone in which practitioners are able to operate safely. When in doubt, go to a higher level of PPE!

Decontamination

Patients and EMS practitioners may require expeditious, or "hasty," decontamination to decrease exposure to life-threatening substances. All EMS practitioners must be familiar with hasty decontamination procedures that may be executed before the formal hazmat/decontamination team arrives.

Timely and effective decontamination is critical to improving patient outcomes but requires large amounts of resources and trained personnel, including the following:

- *Site security*: These practitioners ensure contaminated patients do not wander into "clean" areas.
- *Hot zone (direct threat) medical staff*: These practitioners provide immediate medical care to manage life threats, including tourniquet application, performance of basic airway maneuvers, and administration of chemical agent antidotes before decontamination when feasible.
- *Sufficient decontamination teams to maintain a sustainable work–rest cycle*: Performing decontamination in full PPE can be physically exhausting, particularly in warm ambient temperatures.

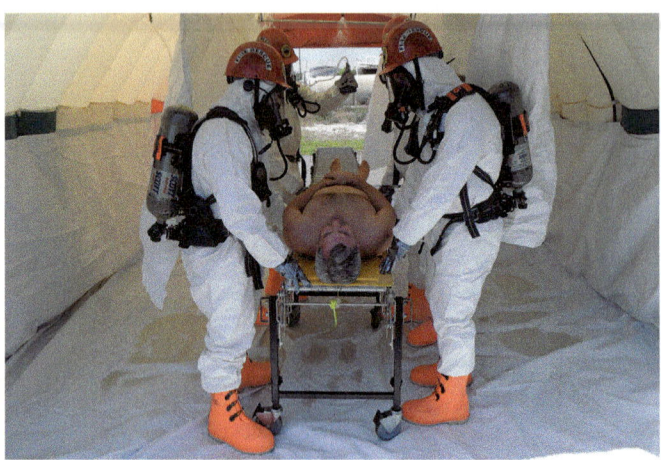

Figure 7-3 Decontamination from nerve agents.
© Jones & Bartlett Learning. Photographed by Glen E. Ellman.

vapor or gases does not require decontamination to prevent secondary contamination, although the victim's clothing should be removed in those cases. Note that before setting up a decontamination zone, a sweep for secondary devices should be performed.

When planning for and setting up a decontamination area, EMS practitioners should consider the following:

- Privacy for all patients or practitioners required to disrobe
- Warm water (when possible) for irrigation and showering
- A suitable substitute for clothing after decontamination
- An approach to assuring victims that their personal belongings will be secure until a final disposition is made regarding their return or necessary disposal
- Means of appropriately disposing of wastewater, if practical

Hot Zone (Direct Threat) Medical Care

Medical care in the hot zone includes interventions to address life threats:

- Tourniquets
- Simple airway maneuvers
- Chemical agent antidotes

Designated Decontamination Areas/Corridors

Decontamination procedures in the field must be performed in designated decontamination areas/corridors, typically upwind and uphill of the affected area when conditions allow (**Figure 7-3**). Known exposure to only

Two-Step Process

Decontamination is a two-step process. The first step involves the removal of all clothing, jewelry, and shoes, which are then bagged, tagged, and secured for later identification. These items may serve as evidence in incident investigation. They may be returned to the owner if successfully decontaminated. The simple act of removing clothing removes the majority of contamination. Any remaining solid contaminant should be carefully brushed away, and any liquid contamination should be blotted off.

The second step involves washing the skin surfaces with water or with water and a mild detergent to remove all substances from the skin. It is important to perform decontamination systematically to avoid missing areas of contaminated skin. When washing, pay special attention to skin folds, axillae, the groin, buttocks, and feet because contaminants can collect in these areas and may be overlooked. Remove contact lenses from the eyes, and irrigate the mucous membranes with copious amounts of water or saline, especially if the patient is symptomatic. Avoid using harsh detergents or bleach solutions on the skin, and scrub gently, as chemically or physically aggravating the skin may contribute to increased absorption of the offending agent. Contain runoff water to keep it from entering irrigation or sewer systems. Use small wading pools or commercially purchased containers to house runoff particles and water.

Take care during the primary decontamination process to ensure that the hazardous material has been completely removed. Secondary decontamination should be performed at the receiving facility to ensure that remnants of the contaminants are removed. After the incident, properly dispose of contaminated clothing. Thoroughly decontaminate rescue and transport vehicles.

Ambulatory vs. Nonambulatory Patients

Ambulatory patients should be able to perform their own decontamination under instruction from EMS practitioners. Nonambulatory patients, and those unable to understand the directions of practitioners, will require the assistance of EMS practitioners properly outfitted with the appropriate PPE to decontaminate patients horizontally (on a litter). After the patient has been decontaminated, a method must be in place for documenting that the patient has undergone decontamination. At this point, asymptomatic victims are not released but are observed to note whether signs of toxicity occur or reoccur, indicating incomplete decontamination.

Situational Awareness in Hazmat Disasters

Situational awareness is critical in ensuring the safety of EMS practitioners. Be aware of the following:

- Control zones may be dynamic.
- Scene safety may be dynamic.
- Secondary contamination may be a constant issue.

Chemical Disasters

Many scenarios can expose EMS practitioners to chemical agents, including industrial incidents, motor vehicle collisions, spilled tanker trucks or railway cars, unearthed military ordnance, or intentional attacks. According to a 2023 analysis of data collected by the EPA and nonprofit groups that track chemical accidents in the United States, accidental releases (e.g., train derailments, truck crashes, pipeline ruptures, industrial plant leaks and spills) occur regularly across the country, possibly as often as once every 2 days.

Classification of Chemical Agents and Toxidromes

Different chemical agents could be involved in a disaster: cyanides, nerve agents, lung toxicants, vesicants, incapacitating agents, lacrimating agents, and vomiting agents (**Table 7-3**). The constellation of clinical signs and symptoms suggesting exposure to certain chemicals or toxins is called a **toxidrome**. Some examples of toxidromes associated with chemical exposures are irritant/corrosive, anticholinergic, cholinergic, anesthetic/sedative, convulsant, knockdown, and **blister agent/vesicant** (**Table 7-4**). If the offending agent is properly identified, or if its identity is suggested by the toxidrome or clinical presentation, therapy specific to the agent may be delivered. Initial interventions will often focus on the management of symptoms such as seizures, secretions, or respiratory distress. Cyanide and nerve agent victims are examples of patients who can benefit from agent-specific antidote therapy.

Severity and Symptoms of Exposure

Several factors determine the severity of a person's reaction to a hazmat exposure, including the type of hazardous material, its chemical components, the route of entry, and the individual's general health. Some signs and symptoms appear immediately, whereas others may be delayed, making it difficult to obtain an accurate patient clinical history. Practitioners should be alert for the following:

- Respiratory distress, dyspnea, and chest tightness
- Nausea and vomiting
- Diarrhea
- Excessive salivation and drooling
- Tingling and numbness of the extremities
- Altered mentation (including seizures)
- Skin discoloration

Table 7-3 Classification of Chemical Agents

Type of Chemical Agent	Examples
Cyanides (blood agents or asphyxiants)	Hydrogen cyanide*, cyanogen chloride
Nerve agents	Tabun (GA), sarin (GB), soman (GD), cyclosarin (GF), VX, some agricultural pesticides
Lung toxicants (choking or pulmonary agents)	Chlorine, phosgene, diphosgene, ammonia
Vesicants (blistering agents)	Sulfur mustard, lewisite
Incapacitating agents	BZ (3-quinuclidinyl benzilate)
Lacrimating agents (riot-control agents)	CN and CS (tear gas agents), oleoresin capsicum (OC or pepper spray)
Vomiting agents**	Adamsite

*Remember that every structure fire releases hydrogen cyanide.

**For vomiting agents, treat the patient's symptoms. The airway needs to stay clear and open. Maintain hydration and electrolyte balances. Do not try to stop the patient's vomiting, because you want the agent to exit the body.

© National Association of Emergency Medical Technicians (NAEMT)

Table 7-4 Toxidromes Associated with Chemical Agents

Toxidrome	Signs/Symptoms	Chemical Agents
Irritant/corrosive	Cough, wheezing, and skin/mucous membrane irritation or inflammation from corrosive acids/bases	Hydrogen fluoride
Anticholinergic	Dilated pupils, confusion, dryness with reduced sweating, temperature elevation	Scopolamine, BZ, tricyclic antidepressants
Cholinergic	Salivation, lacrimation, urination, "leaking all over"	Pesticides, nerve agents (sarin [GB], soman [GD], tabun [GA], VX, and fourth-generation agents [FGAs])
Sedative/anesthetic	Decreased level of consciousness, respiratory depression	Opioids, benzodiazepine
Asphyxiant	Shortness of breath, chest pain, dysrhythmias, syncope, seizures, coma, and death	Cyanide, carbon monoxide
Convulsant	Seizures	Hydrazine, tetramethylenedisulfotetramine (TETS), picrotoxin, strychnine
Knockdown	Asphyxia, decreased level of consciousness, cardiorespiratory effects	Ammonia, chlorine, phosgene
Blister agent/vesicant	Dermal burns, mucosal and dermal irritation, pain, upper and lower airway effects	Lewisite, sulfur mustard, nitrogen mustard

© National Association of Emergency Medical Technicians (NAEMT)

Type of Exposure

Oral and Inhalation

OSHA, along with the EPA and the National Institute for Occupational Safety and Health (NIOSH), has used animal studies to ascertain the exposure levels considered dangerous for each type of hazardous material. This level is expressed using metrics known as the lethal dose, 50% (LD50), and the lethal concentration, 50% (LC50). The LD50 is the level of oral or dermal exposure dose that kills 50% of an exposed animal population in 2 weeks. The LC50 is the air concentration of an agent that kills 50% of the exposed animal population. LD50 applies to hazardous materials when swallowed or absorbed through the skin, whereas LC50 applies to toxic agents when inhaled.

Exposure to agents with low water solubility can seriously damage lung tissue, resulting in irreversible pulmonary edema and long-term chronic lung disease. Exposure to agents with high water solubility, such as ammonia, causes only benign symptoms in the upper airway because such agents are absorbed in the mucous membranes before reaching the lungs. The patient will complain of eye irritation, skin burns, respiratory tract irritation, and a nonproductive cough.

On your initial physical assessment, identify and manage any increased work of breathing. If the patient is wheezing, administer bronchodilators such as albuterol. Give fluids and vasopressors for hypotension. Because of the potential for pulmonary edema, monitor IV fluids closely to avert fluid overload. Once you have completed decontamination protocols, initiate routine supportive care.

Ingestion

Ingestion of hazardous materials is not common and is typically associated with intentional poisoning. However, it can occur if decontamination is not thorough or a hazardous material is poorly labeled. Gastric irritation, including nausea, vomiting, and abdominal pain, is common.

Injection

Injection of a hazardous material may occur intentionally or inadvertently when a practitioner administers a medication to a patient with a contaminated needle. However, penetration through contaminated skin tissue can allow the toxic substance to be absorbed by the body as well, where it may damage organs. The liver metabolizes many injected substances, and this can result in debilitating damage. Identifying a patient's or clinician's risk for this route of exposure is essential in preventing contamination.

Primary and Secondary Contamination

Emergency practitioners can be exposed to chemical agents at the disaster site's release point (primary contamination). **Primary contamination** occurs in the hot zone. Gases, vapors, liquids, solids, and aerosols can all play a role in primary contamination.

EMS practitioners can also be exposed to the chemical agent after it has been carried away from the point of origin, whether by a victim, another EMS practitioner, or a piece of contaminated equipment or debris. This is referred to as **secondary contamination**. Secondary contamination generally occurs in the warm zone, although it may happen at more remote locations if the exposed victim self-evacuates. Solids and liquids (and sometimes aerosols) generally contribute to secondary contamination. Gases and vapors do not typically play a role in secondary contamination because they cause injury by inhalation of the substance and do not deposit on the skin. However, vapors can become trapped in clothing and then off-gas to potentially expose others to the hazard.

Volatility of the Chemical Agent

The volatility of a chemical agent plays a significant role in the risk of secondary contamination. The **volatility** of a substance is the likelihood that the substance (solid or liquid) will vaporize into a gaseous form at room temperature. Highly volatile substances easily convert into gas at room temperature. More volatile substances are considered "less persistent," meaning long-lasting physical contamination is unlikely because the substance will vaporize. These chemical agents will readily disperse and be carried away by the wind. Less volatile substances are considered "more persistent." These substances do not vaporize or do so at a very slow rate, thereby remaining on exposed surfaces for a long time, increasing the risk of secondary contamination. For example, the nerve agent sarin is a nonpersistent agent and evaporates at about the same rate as water, so upon release, the liquid would not be expected to stay in the environment for a long time. By contrast, the nerve agent VX is an organophosphate that is a very persistent agent. It evaporates at the same rate as light motor oil and would be expected to stay in the environment for days to weeks, depending on environmental factors.

Specialized Decontamination Agents

Specialized decontamination agents, including Reactive Skin Decontamination Lotion (commonly referred to as RSDL), fuller's earth, and various other products, contain

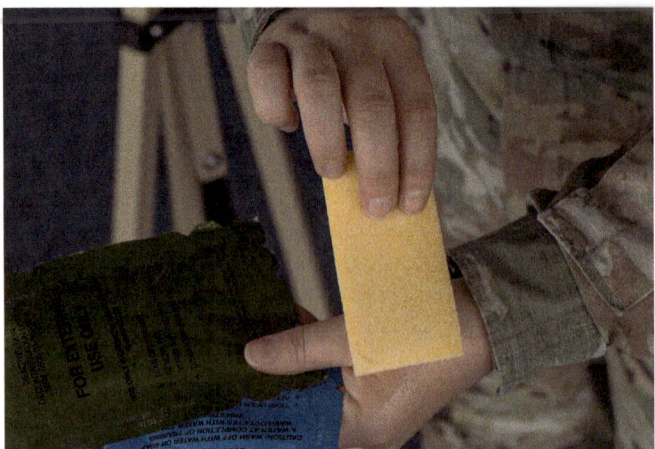

Figure 7-4 Reactive Skin Decontamination Lotion (RSDL).
Courtesy of Airman 1st Class John Wright, U.S. Air Force

active ingredients that may neutralize hazardous chemical agents before they can be fully absorbed through the skin (**Figure 7-4**). The exact mechanism of action and application procedures vary by product. Still, in general, they are incorporated as part of the skin decontamination process. They are used in place of or in addition to traditionally used soap-and-water or diluted sodium hypochlorite (bleach) solutions. Lab and animal models have suggested that these specialized decontamination agents can reduce systemic toxicity and improve survival. EMS agencies should consider adding one or more of these products to their decontamination setup.

EMS Considerations in the Management of Chemical Disasters

After ensuring the scene's safety, EMS practitioners must first administer life-sustaining interventions in the hot (direct threat) zone. The victims then undergo decontamination. Once the victim has been properly decontaminated, EMS practitioners can focus on care of patients with signs and symptoms of exposure to a hazardous substance that has not yet been identified. Evaluating the presenting signs and symptoms and whether they are improving or progressing is important. Patients with worsening clinical findings likely had incomplete cleansing of the contaminant and should undergo repeat decontamination to ensure complete removal.

A repeat primary survey should be performed to determine what other life-sustaining interventions may be immediately required. It is important to note that practitioners often must initiate supportive therapy without knowing the specific chemical cause of the injury. A secondary assessment may then assist in identifying

symptom constellations (toxidromes) that indicate the nature of the chemical agent and suggest a specific antidote.

Chemical Asphyxiants

In contrast to simple asphyxiants (e.g., carbon dioxide, nitrogen gas) that displace oxygen to cause hypoxemia, chemical asphyxiants (e.g., carbon monoxide, cyanide, hydrogen sulfide) interfere with the electron transport chain or other cellular processes and cause hypoxemia not responsive to increased oxygen levels. Exposure to chemical asphyxiants can occur through inhalation, absorption, or ingestion.

One of the most common asphyxiants is hydrogen cyanide, which carries the military designation AC. Notable for its bitter almond-like odor when found in a solid form, cyanide can also be a liquid or a colorless gas. It is often used to treat metals and is a by-product of gas combustion. Cyanide is also very commonly encountered during structural fires because of burning plastics and other materials. A significant level of cyanide is present in as many as 35% of domestic fire victims, making it the most common cause of cyanide poisoning in developed countries. Another chemical asphyxiant used as an agent of warfare is cyanogen chloride, which carries the military designation CK.

Cyanide Toxicity in Structural Fires

Structural fires are a relatively common occurrence, and can be expected following a disaster. EMS practitioners should consider cyanide toxicity in anyone rescued from a fire given any of the following circumstances:

- Person was exposed to fire or smoke in an enclosed area.
- Person has soot around the mouth, nose, or back of the mouth.
- Person shows altered mental status (e.g., confusion, disorientation).

Supportive therapy is important, including high-concentration oxygen delivery, correction of hypotension with fluids or vasopressors, and management of seizures. Assessment of respiratory and cardiovascular status is the key to determining treatment interventions. Routine medical care includes providing supplemental oxygen, administering IV therapy, and monitoring for cardiac dysrhythmias. Cyanide toxicity requires the administration of a cyanide antidote such as hydroxocobalamin.

Hydroxocobalamin is the preferred field antidote for cyanide poisoning because it is easy to use; involves a single medication administration; and, unlike prior antidote kits, does not create an intermediate chemical that is itself a poison. Modern cyanide antidote kits contain IV hydroxocobalamin. If seizure activity occurs, give benzodiazepines. Pulse oximetry readings do not reflect oxygen delivery to cells in cases of chemical asphyxiant exposure.

If the contaminant is a known liquid, initiate the decontamination process immediately. The initial medical interventions are stabilizing the airway, breathing, and circulation and treating presenting signs and symptoms. Give hydroxocobalamin to patients with cyanide toxicity. The cobalt within hydroxocobalamin binds cyanide to form cyanocobalamin or active vitamin B_{12}. The kidneys then excrete cyanocobalamin. Administration of hydroxocobalamin is associated with deep-red to purple staining of body excretions (urine) and secretions and interferes with some colorimetric laboratory studies, including chemistries, for several days. Refer to local protocols, as some EMS agencies will attempt to draw blood tubes for hospital use prior to giving Cyanokit (**Figure 7-5**), but not at the expense of delaying administration.

Nerve Agents

The most toxic agents in chemical warfare are **nerve agents**. These agents disrupt nerve transmission in the

Treatment of Chemical Asphyxiant Exposure

- Remove patients from suspected asphyxiant sources (e.g., carbon monoxide, cyanide, hydrogen sulfide). Give activated charcoal for liquid or solid cyanide ingestion.
- Open the airway. Consider orotracheal or nasotracheal intubation if the patient is unconscious, has severe pulmonary edema, is in severe respiratory distress, or is apneic.
- Provide positive-pressure ventilation with a bag-mask device as needed.
- Do not induce vomiting.
- Monitor for pulmonary edema and treat as necessary.
- Monitor cardiac rhythm and treat dysrhythmias as necessary.
- Establish IV access and infuse crystalloids at 30 mL/h. For hypotension with signs of hypovolemia, give fluid cautiously. Consider vasopressors, per local protocol, if the patient is hypotensive with a normal fluid volume. Watch for signs of fluid overload.
- Administer a cyanide antidote per local protocol for symptomatic patients with cyanide or hydrogen sulfide exposure.
- Treat seizures per local protocol (diazepam/lorazepam/midazolam).
- For eye contamination, immediately flush the eyes with water. Continuously irrigate each eye with normal saline during transport.
- Pulse oximetry readings may not be accurate in these exposures.
- Hyperbaric oxygen may be required for optimal treatment.

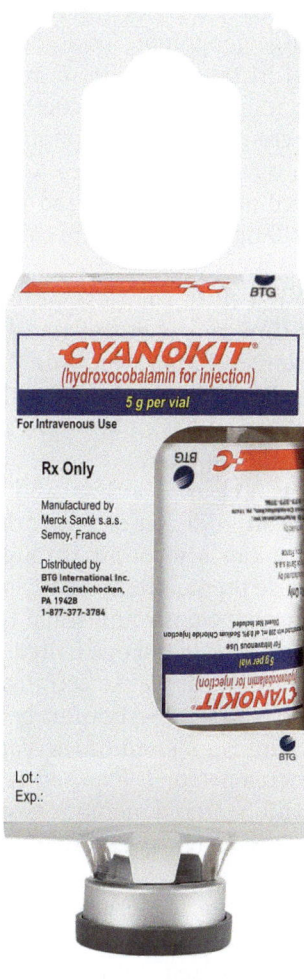

Figure 7-5 Cyanokit.
CYANOKIT is a registered trademark of SERB Sàrl, licensed to BTG International Inc

central and peripheral nervous systems by inhibiting ace-tylcholinesterase, exciting the cholinergic response, and overstimulating the parasympathetic nervous system. Although minimal exposure has no long-term devastating results, high amounts and long duration of exposure are associated with high mortality and morbidity rates. Nerve agents are similar to organophosphates but much more potent and destructive.

Nerve agents can also be classified as G and V agents. The G agents include tabun (GA), sarin (GB), soman (GD), and cyclohexyl methylphosphonofluoridate (GF). Developed in the United Kingdom, VX is the most common V agent. G agents are very volatile, limited-action, colorless liquids. When aerosolized or released into warm environments or closed buildings, they become more volatile. V liquids are usually not volatile and are longer acting.

Sarin (GB) is colorless, odorless, and tasteless in its liquid state. It can infiltrate waterways and reach toxic levels in drinking water or water used for bathing. Sarin can also be converted to a vapor and released into the air, contaminating large geographic areas. People exposed to sarin complain of irritated eyes, nose, mouth, throat, or mucous membranes; cough; headache; increased saliva-tion; abdominal cramping; and respiratory distress with wheezing. Symptoms begin minutes to hours after exposure. This nerve agent was released in a 1995 Tokyo subway attack, killing 12 people and causing more than 5,000 people to seek medical care.

Soman (GD) is a clear, colorless, tasteless liquid with a camphor odor similar to mentholated rubs and cough drops. More volatile than sarin, this liquid provokes symptoms within seconds or minutes rather than hours after exposure. Signs and symptoms are similar to those associated with sarin exposure.

Tabun (GA) is a clear, colorless, and tasteless liquid with a minimal fruity odor. It can vaporize and thus be inhaled. Exposure can also occur through ingestion or absorption. Because the liquid mixes easily with water, it can be ingested, causing gastrointestinal (GI) discomfort. Absorption can cause skin and eye irritation. If the liquid remains on clothing, it can cause secondary contamination of those who touch it. Symptoms begin within seconds when a person is exposed to the vapor and within several hours when a person is exposed to tabun in liquid form. Patients exhibit altered mentation, seizures, watery eyes, cough, and excessive sweating. Cardiac dysrhythmias sometimes occur.

VX, a V agent, is an odorless, slightly amber liquid. This liquid is more toxic when inhaled or absorbed through the skin than when ingested. It mixes easily with water, causing abdominal discomfort when ingested. Signs and symptoms appear within seconds or hours of exposure and are like those provoked by other nerve agents. Victims may have muscle twitching and miosis.

Recognizing Nerve Agent Poisoning

SLUDGEM		Killer Bs	
S	Salivation	B	Bronchospasm
L	Lacrimation	B	Bronchorrhea
U	Urination	B	Bradycardia
D	Defecation		
G	Gastrointestinal upset		
E	Emesis		
M	Miosis		

Unrecognized and untreated, the twitching can progress to status epilepticus and be difficult to stop.

The liquid state of nerve agents makes them a risk for secondary contamination from contact with contaminated clothes, skin, and other objects because these chemicals can stay on clothing 30 to 40 minutes after exposure. Management of nerve agent poisoning includes life-sustaining care prior to decontamination, decontamination, primary survey, administration of antidotes, supportive therapy (including airway, breathing, and circulation support), and continual blood pressure monitoring. Cardiac dysrhythmias should be managed per protocols.

The mnemonics SLUDGEM and Killer Bs can help rescuers identify presenting symptoms of nerve agent poisoning. Symptoms improve after sufficient quantities of antidotes are administered. The three therapeutic medications for managing nerve agent poisoning are atropine, pralidoxime chloride, and benzodiazepines. Older-generation nerve agent autoinjector antidote kits, known as Mark 1 antidote kits, contained separate atropine and pralidoxime autoinjectors. Newer DuoDote kits combine the two medications in one autoinjector. If seizures develop, diazepam or lorazepam IM should be administered (**Figure 7-6**).

EMS practitioners face several challenges when confronted with nerve agent poisoning. Nerve agent poisoning may be initially misinterpreted as an opioid toxidrome. Ventilation and oxygenation of the patient may be difficult because of bronchoconstriction and copious secretions. The patient will likely require frequent suctioning.

Pulmonary Agents/Lung Toxicants

Poisonous gases, known as pulmonary agents or lung toxicants, threaten the safety of first responders and prehospital personnel. These gases, which include chlorine,

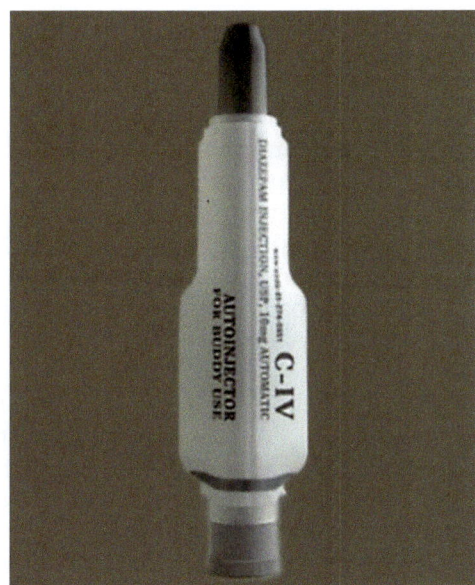

Figure 7-6 Convulsant Antidote for Nerve Agents (CANA).
Courtesy of the USDHHS Radiation Emergency Medical Management

phosgene, and anhydrous ammonia, are found throughout the community and transportation routes, can sometimes be easily obtained, and can quickly contaminate victims through inhalation.

Chlorine is a yellow-green gas with a slight odor that some describe as a combination of pepper and pineapple. It is commonly found in plastics and solvent manufacturing plants. When pressurized, chlorine easily vaporizes into a gas. Chlorine can be inhaled, absorbed through the skin, or ingested if contaminated in water. Signs and symptoms include eye and throat irritation, burns from skin exposure, and respiratory distress caused by inhalation. Severe respiratory complications such as pulmonary edema become evident within 20 to 24 hours of exposure.

Phosgene (CG) appears in gaseous form as a gray-white cloud with the vague odor of freshly baled hay. This agent is commonly found in pesticides, pharmaceuticals, and dyes. Another potential source of phosgene gas is the heating of Freon, which occurs when soldering refrigeration pipes. When cooled, it converts to a liquid. When released into the air, it vaporizes quickly. Early symptoms of exposure may be minimal, as phosgene is far less irritating to mucosal membranes than chlorine, for instance. However, delayed pulmonary injury and edema may develop 24 or more hours later and can be fatal. The agent can cause significant cardiovascular compromise and hypotension. If the exposure is not identified and managed, death can occur within a few days. Physical exertion worsens and intensifies the pulmonary injury, so the patient should be kept calm.

Anhydrous ammonia is a colorless gas commonly found in agricultural settings and used as fertilizer. Industrial factories use this gas for cooling and freezing foods such as meat and poultry. Anhydrous ammonia is considered volatile and forms a white cloud when present in high concentrations. Symptoms occur within several hours of exposure. Ammonia irritates the eyes, skin, respiratory tract, and GI tract. It can cause eye and skin irritation and burning sensations. If ingested or inhaled, symptoms include nausea, vomiting, abdominal pain, burning, and swelling of the lips, mouth, and throat. Patients succumb to overwhelming asphyxiation.

Unfortunately, no antidote exists for these chemicals. Management of lung toxicants includes removal of the patient from the offending agent, decontamination with copious irrigation (in case of solid, liquid, or aerosol exposure, especially for ammonia), primary survey, and supportive therapy, which will likely require interventions to maximize ventilation and oxygenation. Eye irritation can be managed with copious irrigation using normal saline.

Vesicant Agents

In a mass-casualty incident with multiple vesicant agents, EMS practitioners must consider an intentional event and ensure that law enforcement is informed.

Sulfur mustard is an oily, clear yellow-brown liquid that can be aerosolized by a bomb blast or sprayer. Its low volatility allows it to persist on surfaces for a week or more. This persistence allows for easy secondary contamination. The agent is absorbed through the skin and mucous membranes, resulting in direct cellular damage within 3 to 5 minutes of the exposure (**Figure 7-7**). However, clinical symptoms and signs may take 1 to 12 hours (usually 4 to 6 hours) after exposure to develop. The delayed onset of symptoms often makes it difficult for the victim to recognize that the exposure occurred, increasing the potential for secondary contamination. Warm, moist skin increases the likelihood of skin absorption, making the groin and axillary regions particularly susceptible. The eyes, skin, and upper airways can develop a range of findings, from erythema and edema to vesicle development to full-thickness necrosis. Upper airway involvement can result in cough and bronchospasm. High-dose exposures can result in nausea, vomiting, and bone marrow suppression.

Management for sulfur mustard exposure involves decontamination using soap and water, completing a primary survey, and providing supportive therapy. No antidote exists for the effects of mustard agents. Pulmonary bronchoconstriction may benefit from nebulized beta agonists. Skin wounds should be treated as burns with local wound care. It is important to note that because the cellular damage from sulfur mustard occurs within

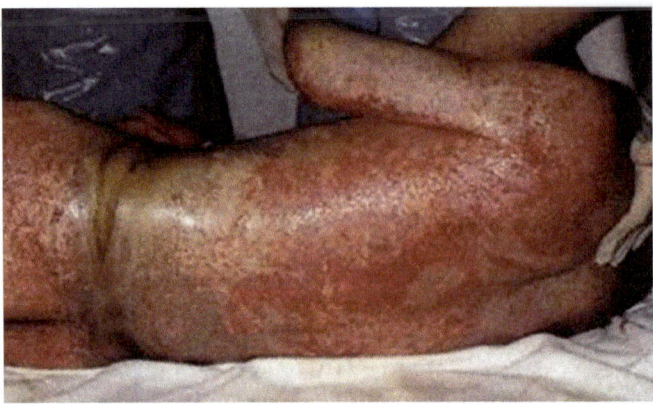

Figure 7-7 Skin damage caused by exposure to sulfur mustard.
Courtesy of Dr. Saeed Keshavarz/Research Center of Chemical Injuries/IRAN

several minutes of the exposure, decontamination will not change the clinical course of the exposed patient. It is primarily intended to prevent inadvertent cross contamination. Eyes and skin should be decontaminated with copious amounts of water as soon as exposure is recognized to minimize further agent absorption and prevent secondary contamination. The fluid in resulting vesicles and blisters is not a source of secondary contamination.

Lewisite has a similar constellation of symptoms, but the onset of action is much quicker than sulfur mustard, resulting in immediate pain and irritation to the eyes, skin, and respiratory tract. Unlike sulfur mustard, lewisite does not cause bone marrow suppression. Also unique to this agent is "lewisite shock," resulting from intravascular volume depletion secondary to capillary leakage. As with sulfur mustard, prehospital management of patients exposed to lewisite involves decontamination, a primary survey, and supportive care. British anti-lewisite is an antidote available for the in-hospital treatment of patients who have been exposed to lewisite. It is administered intravenously for patients with hypovolemic shock or pulmonary symptoms. Applied topically, British anti-lewisite ointment has been reported to prevent mucous membrane and skin injury. Practitioners should be careful to avoid contact with the fluid inside skin blisters caused by lewisite, as it may contain toxic arsenic compounds and active lewisite or dangerous breakdown products.

Transport Considerations

Contaminated patients should not be transported until they have been decontaminated. Transporting contaminated patients results in cross contamination of the vehicle and personnel, thus taking them out of service until they have been decontaminated. This compromised EMS response may prolong the scene time and management of ill or injured patients. This same concern about not transporting contaminated patients applies to air medical services.

EMS practitioners should bring patients to an appropriate medical treatment facility for further evaluation and management. Transporting to the optimal facility is particularly important because some chemical toxic effects may not become apparent for 8 to 24 hours. Communities may identify preferred hospitals for the management of chemical casualties. Such facilities may be more capable of managing these patients by virtue of specialized training or availability of critical care services and specific antidotes.

EMS systems should keep a detailed count of all patients transported from the scene and their destination hospitals. Nearby EDs may become overwhelmed by ambulatory, self-evacuated, self-transported patients. Of the 640 patients presenting to one hospital in Tokyo after the sarin incident, 541 arrived without EMS assistance. Hospitals closest to the event will likely receive the largest number of ambulatory patients. These factors should be considered in determining the destination of patients transported via ambulance.

Establish centralized communications with area hospitals early in the incident and with a transportation officer to help route ambulances and guide destinations.

Radiologic/Nuclear Disasters

Radiation incidents have the potential to cause large numbers of both immediate and longer-term casualties. The Chernobyl disaster of 1986 was responsible for 116,500 to 125,000 exposed casualties. The Fukushima nuclear power plant in Japan was seriously damaged after an earthquake and tsunami in 2011, resulting in the destruction of several reactors and the release of radiation into the environment. It will take years and even decades before the health impact of this incident on the surrounding population and environment can be fully evaluated.

Radiation disasters can generate fear and confusion in both victims and EMS practitioners. Familiarization with the hazard and management principles will help ensure an appropriate response and reduce panic and disorder.

Types of Ionizing Radiation

Nuclear radiation comprises particles and energy released when atoms break up (fission) or combine (fusion). Ionizing radiation refers to radiation (alpha, beta, gamma, and neutron) with sufficient energy to strip electrons from atoms or molecules. Essentially, all types of radiation from the atomic nucleus are ionizing.

Alpha particles (protons and neutrons) are relatively large and cannot penetrate even a few layers of the skin. They travel only a few feet and can be blocked by a simple barrier such as paper. Intact skin or a uniform offers adequate protection from external contamination emitting alpha particles. They present a significant biohazard only when radioactive material is inhaled or ingested.

Beta particles (electrons) are smaller and faster than alpha particles and thus can travel farther, penetrating tissue to a depth of about 8 mm. They can cause significant burns to the skin's surface, although the burns are not usually visible immediately after exposure. Because clothing effectively shields covered areas, the primary danger is to the exposed skin. Standard skin-cleansing procedures remove most of the contamination from beta particles. The only means of detection of beta particles is a radiation-sensing instrument called a Geiger-Müller counter, which all hospitals should have. If exposure continues, significant exposure to gamma radiation can occur, because most radioisotopes decay by emitting beta radiation followed by gamma emission.

Gamma rays are photons emitted from the nucleus of the atom. They are electromagnetic waves that travel quickly and penetrate deeply through skin, soft tissue, and bone. Gamma rays are involved in nearly all accidents involving external irradiation. X-rays are relatively lower-energy photons that are occasionally involved in radiation accidents arising from improper use of industrial or medical equipment. Gamma rays are emitted from radioisotopes after beta decay and are the primary cause of **acute radiation syndrome** (phases of this syndrome are outlined in **Table 7-5**). Delayed effects occur in symptom clusters (**Table 7-6**). The U.S. Department of Health and Human Services maintains the Radiation Emergency Medical Management website at https://remm.hhs.gov as a reference for medical professionals.

The fourth form of radiation, neutron radiation, easily penetrates surfaces. It has 20 times the destructive energy of gamma rays and can cause significant damage to body systems. Neutrons are unique. When they are stopped, or "captured," after emission, they cause previously stable atoms to become radioactive. This is the source of radioactive fallout. The surface burst of a thermonuclear weapon instantly vaporizes tons of soil, transforming it by intense neutron bombardment into highly radioactive material. This cloud—the so-called mushroom cloud we associate with the nuclear bomb—rises with the fireball and is carried away by the prevailing winds at high altitudes. Its radioactive particles ultimately descend as fallout. A nuclear reactor harnesses this same powerful form of radiation by creating a controlled, sustained neutron chain reaction to generate energy.

Some gamma exposure also occurs with neutron exposure. Quantifying the radioactive material generated by neutron irradiation helps estimate neutron exposure and, sometimes indirectly, the dose of gamma radiation. The radioactivity generated is primarily sodium-24, which can be detected by a Geiger-Müller counter or in a blood sample. If neutron exposure is suspected, clinicians should save and refrigerate all patient feces and urine. In addition, clinicians should save all clothing, especially items containing metal parts such as belt buckles, for analysis of neutron-induced radioisotopes.

Measuring Ionizing Radiation

Whole-body exposure to ionizing radiation is measured in terms of the gray (Gy). The rad (radiation absorbed dose) was a familiar dose unit that was replaced by the gray; 1 Gy equals 100 rad. The rem (radiation equivalent-man) describes the dose in rad multiplied by a "quality factor" that takes into account the intrinsic special deposition pattern of different types of radiation. This term has been replaced with the sievert (Sv); 1 Sv equals 100 rem. Assessing a patient exposed to ionizing radiation requires determining the dose of gray they absorbed. The greater the dose of gray absorbed, the greater the potential for serious illness and injury.

Radiation affects rapidly dividing cells most readily, resulting in injury to the bone marrow and GI tract where high cell turnover rates occur. Higher doses can affect the CNS directly. The dose of whole-body exposure determines the medical consequences of the exposure. Patients receiving up to 1 Gy of whole-body irradiation would typically not exhibit signs of injury. At 1 to 2 Gy, fewer than one-half of patients will develop nausea and vomiting, many will subsequently develop leukopenia (decreased white blood cell count), and deaths will be minimal. Most victims receiving greater than 2 Gy will become ill and require hospitalization; at greater than 6 Gy, mortality becomes high. At doses greater than 30 Gy, neurologic signs manifest and death is most likely.

Disaster Scenarios

Exposure to ionizing radiation and radioactive contamination may result from several different scenarios, including the following:

- Nuclear weapon, whether high-grade or an improvised low-yield device
- A dirty bomb or radiologic dispersion device, in which there is no nuclear detonation, but rather conventional explosives are detonated to disperse a radionuclide (radioactive material)

Table 7-5 Phases of Acute Radiation Syndrome

Feature	Effects of Whole-Body Irradiation from External Radiation or Internal Absorption by Dose Range in Rad (1 Rad = 1 cGy; 100 Rad = 1 Gy)					
	0–100	100–200	200–600	600–800	800–3000	> 3000
Prodromal Phase						
Nausea, vomiting	None	5%–50%	50%–100%	75%–100%	90%–100%	100%
Time of onset	N/A	3–6 hr	2–4 hr	1–2 hr	< 1 hr	N/A
Duration	N/A	< 24 hr	< 24 hr	< 48 hr	48 hr	N/A
Lymphocyte count	Unaffected	Minimally decreased	< 1,000 at 24 hr	< 500 at 24 hr	Decreases within hours	Decreases within minutes
CNS function	No impairment	No impairment	Routine task performance Cognitive impairment for 6–20 hr	Simple, routine task performance Cognitive impairment for > 24 hr	Rapid incapacitation; may have a lucid interval of several hours	
Latent Phase						
No symptoms	> 2 wk	7–15 days	0–7 days	0–2 days	None	None
Manifest Illness						
Signs/symptoms	None	Moderate leukopenia	Severe leukopenia, purpura, hemorrhage, pneumonia, hair loss after 300 rad		Diarrhea, fever, electrolyte disturbance	Convulsions, ataxia, tremor, lethargy
Time of onset	N/A	> 2 wk	2 days–4 wk		1–3 days	1–3 days
Critical period	N/A	None	4–6 wk; greatest potential for effective medical intervention		2–14 days	1–46 hr
Organ system	None	N/A	Hematopoietic; respiratory (mucosal) systems		GI tract Mucosal systems	CNS
Hospitalization duration	0%	< 5% 45–60 days	90% 60–90 days	100% 100+ days	100% Weeks to months	100% Days to weeks
Mortality	None	Minimal	Low with aggressive therapy	High	Very high; significant neurologic symptoms indicate lethal dose	

Abbreviations: CNS, central nervous system; GI, gastrointestinal; hr, hour(s); N/A, not applicable; wk, week(s)

Armed Forces Radiobiology Institute. Medical Management of Radiological Casualties. Armed Forces Radiobiology Institute; 2003.

Table 7-6 Symptom Clusters as Delayed Effects of Radiation Exposure

1	2	3	4
Headache Fatigue Weakness	Anorexia Nausea Vomiting Diarrhea	Partial-thickness and full-thickness skin damage Depilation (hair loss) Ulceration	Lymphopenia Neutropenia Thrombocytopenia Purpura Opportunistic infections

© National Association of Emergency Medical Technicians (NAEMT)

- Sabotage or an incident at a nuclear reactor site
- Transportation incident involving nuclear waste
- Mishandled nuclear waste

Types of Radiologic Weapons

Four types of weapons can cause a radiologic incident:

- A **radiologic dispersal device (RDD)** is a conventional explosive device with radiologic contaminants or a device that can disperse radioactive material. RDDs disperse radioactive material over a large area, causing contamination and internal/external exposures. A terrorist can intentionally detonate such an explosive device as a dirty bomb in a highly populated area. Contamination of humans, animals, buildings, and the environment occurs when radioactive materials such as cobalt-60 and radium-226 are released. The initial blast will cause traumatic injury. If radiologic exposure is not recognized early, prolonged exposure can cause emergent medical problems. Inhalation of radioactive particles can provoke respiratory distress, and ingestion can induce GI discomfort.
- A **radiologic exposure device (RED)** is designed to expose people to radiation only (no contamination). REDs cause smaller, more limited hot zone results than RDDs and external exposures.
- A **radiologic incendiary device (RID)** is a device that pairs fire with radiologic contamination. It is used to delay first responders deliberately and causes internal and external exposures.
- An **improvised nuclear device (IND)** is an illicit nuclear weapon/fabricated nuclear weapon associated with extensive (catastrophic) casualties with multiple types of injuries.

Diagnosing Radiation Exposure

The extent of injury and illness from the initial blast of a radioactive device is related to the duration (time) of exposure, distance from the explosion or blast, and the amount of the person's protection (shielding). Exposed persons may contaminate others if gas, liquid, or dust particles on their bodies or clothing are transferred. First-response clinicians must ascertain accurate information regarding time, distance, and shielding.

Acute radiation syndrome generally follows a predictable pattern after substantial exposure or catastrophic events (see Table 7-5). Individuals may become ill from contaminated sources in the community and may be identified over much longer periods based on specific syndromes (see Table 7-6). Specific syndromes of concern, especially with a 2- to 3-week prior history of nausea and vomiting, include the following:

- Thermal burn–like skin effects without documented thermal exposure
- Immunologic dysfunction with secondary infections
- Tendency to bleed (epistaxis, gingival bleeding, petechiae)
- Marrow suppression (neutropenia, lymphopenia, and thrombocytopenia)
- Depilation (hair loss)

Understanding Radiation Exposure

Exposure may be known and recognized or clandestine and may occur by the following means: (1) large recognized exposures, such as a nuclear bomb or damage to a nuclear power station; (2) small radiation source emitting continuous gamma radiation, producing group or individual chronic intermittent exposures (e.g., radiologic sources from medical treatment devices, environmental pollution, water or food pollution); and (3) internal radiation from absorbed, inhaled, or ingested radioactive material (internal contamination).

Preventing Untoward Effects from Radiation Exposure

None of the typical PPE protects from a high-energy point source of radiation. This type of radiation is encountered during the first minute of a nuclear detonation, in a critical reactor core, or with a high-energy radiation source such as cesium-137. In such situations, the concept of time/distance/shielding is key in preventing untoward effects from radiation exposure. Radiation exposure is minimized by decreasing time in the affected area, increasing distance from a radiation source, and using shielding materials, such as metal or concrete, that will protect against gamma radiation and neutrons.

Dose Rate Meters and Radiation Surveys

EMS practitioners who work in areas of radiation exposure should wear **dose rate** meters or alarms, which measure dose rates of ionizing radiation. Standards exist for acceptable doses of ionizing radiation in the occupational environment under normal and emergency conditions. The practitioners should approach the incident commander or safety officer for guidance on radiation exposure readings and limits. Dose rate meters or alarms prevent practitioners from putting themselves at risk for acute radiation illness or an unacceptably higher cancer incidence. All practitioners who operate in an environment potentially contaminated with radioactive material should also undergo a radiation survey to determine if internal contamination has occurred and active management (if warranted).

Principles of Management and Decontamination

Initial interventions focus on ensuring scene safety and donning appropriate PPE. Practitioners must protect themselves from radioactive contamination by observing, at a minimum, standard precautions, including protective clothing, gloves, and a mask, which are very important to help prevent GI and respiratory exposures. They should avoid direct contact with radioactive materials.

EMS practitioners should medically stabilize patients from their traumatic injuries before considering radiation injuries. They must also evaluate patients for external radiation exposure and contamination. If great enough, an external source of radiation can cause tissue injury, but it does not make the patient radioactive. Patients with even lethal external radiation exposure do not threaten medical staff. Patients who develop nausea, vomiting, or skin erythema within 4 hours of exposure have probably received a high dose of external radiation.

Practitioners should treat radioactive contamination in wounds as dirty and irrigate as soon as possible. They should avoid handling any metallic foreign body. Potassium iodide (KI) is of value in case of radioactive iodine release; however, it is not a general radiation antidote. For a patient with a life-threatening condition, treat and then decontaminate. For a patient with a non-life-threatening condition, decontaminate and then treat.

Patients can become contaminated with radioactive material deposited on their skin or clothing. Note that decontamination during a radiologic event is almost always dry, as washing may lead to contaminated runoff, and dry decontamination is largely effective in removing secondary contamination. The five types of dry decontamination are scraping, adsorbent materials, absorbent materials, vacuuming, and pressurized air. More than 90% of surface contamination can be removed by clothing removal. The remainder can be washed off with soap and water.

Start decontamination with those suspected of contamination by removing clothing and placing it in an airtight container with appropriate radioactive labeling. A whole-body radiation survey should be performed, and a felt-tip marker should mark areas of high radioactivity. Decontamination should try to achieve radiation levels no more than two times the background levels for external contamination. Two whole-body decontamination cycles should be completed, with a radiation survey completed after each. If radiation continues to be higher than two times the background or does not decrease by at least 10%, practitioners should cover the high-radiation area with a waterproof drape and transport the patient to the hospital. A disproportionately high radiation level in an individual patient may be due to internal contamination, radiation shrapnel, or radiation trapped in the outermost layer of the skin. If possible, the nostrils should be swabbed to determine possible levels of inhalation radioactivity.

EMS practitioners should notify the receiving facility of the contamination from the scene to allow for appropriate precautions on arrival. Practitioners should be mindful of the psychological effects of sustaining a sudden, violent injury and illness from the blast. In mass-casualty situations, local medical and response-team resources can easily become overwhelmed. Verbal communication is an important part of the team effort to minimize contamination efficiently and to assess and manage multiple patients effectively.

Transport Considerations

EMS personnel should transport patients to the nearest appropriate medical center that is capable of managing trauma and radiation injuries. All hospitals are required to have a plan for the management of a radiologic emergency, but communities may have identified specific specialty resource institutions that have decontamination facilities, are capable of managing trauma, and have staff trained to deal effectively with possible external or internal radioactive contamination, as well as the complications of whole-body exposure to ionizing radiation. EMS practitioners must coordinate with local law enforcement and the medical examiner regarding plans for contaminated fatalities.

CASE STUDY

Background

You work for a fire-based EMS organization with multiple transport units in an urban setting. You and your partner are working an evening shift during peak call time. Only four ambulances are currently available for emergency calls. Multiple sporting events are taking place in the city tonight, with an anticipated surge of 100,000 people coming into the city for the sporting events alone.

Mutual aid is up to 25 miles away and includes 10 ambulances with ALS capabilities serving an urban setting. Additional mutual aid consists of four suburban communities 10 miles away, with 2 ambulances per community. An ambulance medical bus that can be fully staffed in 30 minutes is in the community. Additionally, air medical services, with two rotor wings and two fixed wings, are in the community.

How many patients could result in an infectious disease/biologic disaster/chemical disaster in this situation?

Given that you have four ambulances available, more than four patients could lead to a need to activate mutual aid resources.

Dispatch

You and your partner are dispatched to a rail station adjacent to three large sporting venues for multiple patients complaining of respiratory symptoms.

On-Scene Actions

Upon arrival, you are the first unit on scene. One practitioner will be incident commander, and the other will serve as the triage officer (until relieved of command or conclusion of the MCI). As you arrive on scene, you find bystanders providing first aid to patients.

LCAN Report

Location: Rapid transit station

- You are staging one block away from the transit station.

Conditions: Clear sunny day

- 30–50 patients
- Multiple transit police officers are on the scene reporting via radio that they have 30–50 people, all coughing, coming out of one of the train platforms.

- Reports indicate that a "cloud" was seen on one of the trains that just arrived. The "cloud" could have been from a chemical dispersal device located on the train.
- People are beginning to panic and run from the transit station.

Actions: Establish command and begin triage.

- Use regional triage system for case study.

Needs: Identify reinforcement needs.

- Additional ambulances and hazmat team should be requested.
- Discuss alternate transport methods that could be used.
- Could the ambulance medical bus (AMBUS) be used in this case? Consider that the time to activate the AMBUS is 30 minutes.

What are your initial concerns based on the dispatch information?

The initial impression begins when the dispatch information is received. Initial concerns include the following:

- Weather
- Number and severity of patients
- Different age groups of patients
- Available resources
- Triage
- Evacuation of the scene
- Special tools/equipment
- Transport decisions

What potential patient populations do you expect?

- Pediatrics
- Adults (including patients who are parents with small children)
- Elderly

How do scene assessment and awareness apply to this case?

Unknown numbers of people concentrated in one area with the same complaints should raise suspicion. The incident should be treated as a disaster or act of terrorism until proven otherwise.

Scene Safety/PPE

What PPE could protect you based on the dispatch information in a chemical disaster, infectious disease outbreak, or biologic disaster?

In this case, PPE should focus on respiratory protection, as it is the primary source of patient complaints. While level A may be the most appropriate, level B or C would be useful and offer minimum protection.

What should you do to access patients in a rapid transit station to prevent further contamination?

- Personal safety is the number one priority. EMS personnel should not place themselves at unnecessary risk without the proper PPE or safety equipment.
- Patients could need protective equipment (such as masks). For example, patients exposed to biologic agents could contaminate additional responders, bystanders, or health care personnel. Providing patients with the appropriate PPE for treatment and transport would be ideal for source control to help prevent contaminating others.

Patient Triage Review

How many patients are expected?

- The 30 to 50 patients on scene could be at various triage levels (green, yellow, red, black).
- Even without severe injuries, all patients will require triage and transport.

Does primary triage change in this case for this many patients?

What type of patient findings do you expect?

- Runny nose and watery eyes
- Small, pinpoint pupils
- Eye pain or blurred vision
- Drooling and excessive sweating
- Cough
- Chest tightness
- Respiratory distress
- Diarrhea
- Nausea, vomiting, and/or abdominal pain
- Increased urination
- Confusion
- Drowsiness
- Weakness
- Headache
- Slow or fast heart rate
- Low or high blood pressure

What treatment options do you have during patient triage?

- Treatment options will be limited to life-sustaining interventions during primary triage.
- Once everyone is triaged, more detailed treatment could begin.
- Discuss initial treatment options per local guidelines and policy.

Are there any barriers to using a triage system in this case?

- There could be potential limitations in accessing patients. Everyone may have the same presentation and complaint, or it may be difficult to separate those affected and those who are not, making it difficult to triage patients in this setting effectively.
- It may be necessary to focus on securing and isolating the incident and then proceed with decontaminating persons within the designated incident perimeter.

Discuss any competing priorities during triage.

- Triage is going to be challenging and will be performed as patients are accessed.
- Discuss the triage systems (e.g., SALT, START) and how they could be applied in this incident.
- It may be necessary to focus on securing and isolating the incident and then proceed with decontaminating persons within the incident perimeter.

Note that primary triage takes place where the patient is found and it should only take a few minutes to triage all the patients.

Patient Evacuation

What complications may occur during evacuation?

EMS personnel must identify the advantages and disadvantages of evacuating patients when planning to move or receive patients to ensure the safe handling of all involved.

- A multipatient transport option, such as an ambulance medical bus, may facilitate the evacuation and transport of stable, noncritical victims.
- Mutual aid will be necessary in this event to assist with evacuation.
- The number of people who will self-evacuate and transport themselves to a health care facility should be considered, and early notification to the hospital should be made as quickly as possible.
- The incident may become a much larger disaster when masses of people begin arriving at area hospitals.

- It is critical to notify health care facilities of the disaster. This could give them time to prepare for the influx of patients and don the appropriate PPE to manage the disaster.

Secondary Triage

In a chemical disaster, selecting a safe location for a **secondary triage**/treatment area could be difficult. Secondary triage is typically performed when the patient arrives at the treatment area or a casualty collection point.

What are the options for secondary triage in this case?

How can patients be prevented from leaving the secondary triage area?

Case Progression

New reports suggest that at least 500 people have been exposed to the agent and have symptoms. The ICS has been initiated, and mutual aid resources from around the area have been activated and are on the way. Federal agency support, including the National Guard, has been requested. Multiple ambulances and the ambulance medical bus are arriving, and you are relieved by a senior officer and asked to integrate with transport. You and your partner are directed to provide medical triage and oversight of multiple noncritical patients transported on a transit bus (20 victims) with two EMTs/firefighters to assist.

What are the treatment priorities?

- Atropine/2-PAM chloride should be administered if available as a chemical nerve agent antidote.

List the equipment you will need on the bus for managing the patients.

- Focus on resource allocation and preparing for the worst-case scenario.
- Bring along several jump bags, oxygen, and antidote medications (atropine in this case).

Transportation

Assess facility options continuously to prevent overwhelming area hospitals, and ensure that patients are transported according to incident command guidance.

What could happen if you were in a rural or suburban area with so many patients?

- Normal transport patterns could be disrupted due to a large influx of patients, bystanders, and media, creating traffic congestion in the area.
- Patients may self-transport to health care facilities, which could lead to further exposure cases.

What additional resources could assist on site?

- Regional medical assistance teams would be beneficial in managing and treating patients on the scene.
- This could assist with preventing further contamination.

CASE WRAP UP

The initial incident was determined to be a sarin nerve agent attack that affected persons on a single train after a dispersal device was activated. Within 7 days of the attack, an estimated 2,500 people reported to various EDs with signs and symptoms consistent with both sarin and anthrax exposure.

Multiple red, yellow, and green triage-level patients were reported:

- Red tags indicated respiratory failure requiring support.
- Yellow tags indicated moderate exposure symptoms.
- Green-tagged patients had minor symptoms, including coughing, and various injuries due to running from the scene.

Authorities determined that a mixed agent dispersal device was activated that contained both sarin and anthrax spores in order to cause short- and long-term incidents and to maximize fatalities. The persons responsible were linked to an international terror organization.

Could something similar occur in your area?

It is important to understand that terrorism can happen anywhere and to anyone. Although the scenario might differ depending on the area, the outcome could be just as catastrophic.

SUMMARY

- Primary contamination is exposure to the chemical agent at its point of release.
- Secondary contamination is exposure to a chemical agent after it has been carried away from the point of origin, whether by a victim, an EMS practitioner, or a piece of contaminated equipment or debris.
- If possible, approach a disaster scene from an uphill, upwind direction if hazardous materials are suspected.
- When approaching a hazmat incident scene, it is important to identify the source of the hazard and the conditions surrounding the incident, such as the integrity of any packages or containers and chemical placards on vehicles, packages, and containers.
- The designation of the zones of operation must consider temperature, wind directions, topography, runoff, spill size, volatility of the material, and occupancy types surrounding the incident.
- Evaluation and management of a patient exposed to a chemical agent involves the initial life-sustaining care before decontamination, decontamination, repeated primary survey to identify immediate lifesaving intervention, secondary assessment to identify a toxidrome, and initiation of therapy based on the toxidrome/agent.
- Patients and EMS practitioners may require expeditious, or "hasty," decontamination to decrease exposure time to various life-threatening substances. All EMS practitioners must be familiar with a hasty decontamination procedure that may be executed before the formal hazmat/decontamination team arrives.
- Radiation exposure is minimized by decreasing time in the affected area, increasing distance from a radiation source, and using metal or concrete shielding.
- Patients can become contaminated with radioactive material deposited on their skin or clothing. Over 90% of surface radiologic contamination can be removed by clothing removal. The remainder can be washed off with soap and water.
- Radioactive contamination in wounds should be treated as dirt and irrigated immediately.
- Note that decontamination during a radiologic event is almost always dry and is largely effective in removing secondary contamination. Washing may lead to contaminated runoff.
- For a patient with a life-threatening condition: treat and then decontaminate.
- For a patient with a non-life-threatening condition: decontaminate and then treat.
- Do not transport contaminated patients until they have been decontaminated.

References and Additional Resources

Carini F. Ohio derailment that spilled toxic chemicals and shook community should raise alarms here. *ecoRI News*. May 5, 2023. https://www.preventionweb.net/news/ohio-derailment-spilled-toxic-chemicals-and-shook-community-should-raise-alarms-here. Accessed July 19, 2023.

Centers for Disease Control and Prevention's Agency for Toxic Substances and Disease Registry. https://www.atsdr.cdc.gov/emergencyresponse/index.html. Accessed December 11, 2023.

Centers for Disease Control and Prevention. Cyanide: exposure, decontamination, treatment. Last reviewed February 7, 2023. https://www.cdc.gov/chemicalemergencies/factsheets/cyanide.html. Accessed July 20, 2023.

Flynn DF, Goans RE. Nuclear terrorism: triage and medical management of radiation and combined-injury casualties. *Surg Clin North Am*. 2006;86(3):601–636.

Greenfield RA, Brown BR, Hutchins JB, et al. Microbiological, biological and chemical weapons of warfare and terrorism. *Am J Med Sci*. 2002;323(6):326–340.

Hogan DE, Kellison T. Nuclear terrorism. *Am J Med Sci*. 2002;323(6):341–349.

Johnson J. Household fires can cause cyanide poisoning—here's what medical professionals can do. BTG Specialty Pharmaceuticals. March 31, 2022. https://btgsp.com/en-us/insights/household-fires-can-cause-cyanide-poisoning-here-s. Accessed July 19, 2023.

McDonough JH, Capacio BR, Shih TM. Treatment of nerve-agent-induced status epilepticus in the nonhuman primate. In: *U.S. Army Medical Defense—Bioscience Review, June 2–7*. U.S. Army Medical Research Institute; 2002.

National Association of Emergency Medical Technicians. *Advanced Medical Life Support*. 3rd ed. Jones & Bartlett Learning; 2021.

National Association of Emergency Medical Technicians. *Prehospital Trauma Life Support*. 10th ed. Jones & Bartlett Learning; 2023.

Okumura T, Takasu N, Ishimatsu S, et al. Report on 640 victims of the Tokyo subway sarin attack. *Ann Emerg Med*. 1996;28(2):129–135.

Reddy SD, Reddy DS. Midazolam as an anticonvulsant antidote for organophosphate intoxication—a pharmacotherapeutic appraisal. *Epilepsia*. 2015;56(6):813–821.

Rotenberg JS, Newmark J. Nerve-agent attacks on children: diagnosis and management. *Pediatrics*. 2003;112:648–658.

Sellstrom A, Cairns S, Barbeschi M. *Report of United Nations Mission to Investigate Allegations of the Use of Chemical Weapons in the Syrian Arab Republic on the Alleged Use of Chemical Weapons in the Ghouta Area of Damascus on 21 August 2013*. United Nations. Published September 16, 2013. https://digitallibrary.un.org/record/756814?ln=en. Accessed January 31, 2022.

Sidell FR, Takafuji ET, Franz DR, eds. *Medical Aspects of Chemical and Biological Warfare, TMM Series. Part 1: Warfare, Weaponry and the Casualty*. Office of the Surgeon General, TMM Publications; 1997.

Tuorinsky SD. *Textbooks of Military Medicine: Medical Aspects of Chemical Warfare*. Borden Institute, Walter Reed Army Medical Center; 2008.

United Nations, Security Council. Organization for the Prohibition of Chemical Weapons–United Nations Joint Investigative Mechanism. *Fourth Report of the Organization for the Prohibition of Chemical Weapons–United Nations Joint Investigative Mechanism*. Published October 21, 2016. http://undocs.org/S/2016/888. Accessed January 31, 2022.

U.S. Army, Medical Research Institute of Chemical Defense. *Medical Management of Chemical Casualties Handbook*. U.S. Army Research Institute; 2000.

U.S. Department of Health and Human Services. CHEMPACK: Chemical Hazards Emergency Medical Management. Updated August 16, 2021. https://chemm.hhs.gov/chempack.htm. Accessed July 20, 2023.

U.S. Department of Health and Human Services. Radiation Emergency Medical Management. https://remm.hhs.gov. Accessed December 11, 2023.

Walter FG, ed. *Advanced HAZMAT Life Support*. 2nd ed. Arizona Board of Regents; 2000.

World Health Organization, International Atomic Energy Agency, United Nations Development Programme. Chernobyl: the true scale of the accident. Published September 5, 2005. https://www.who.int/news/item/05-09-2005-chernobyl-the-true-scale-of-the-accident. Accessed January 31, 2022.

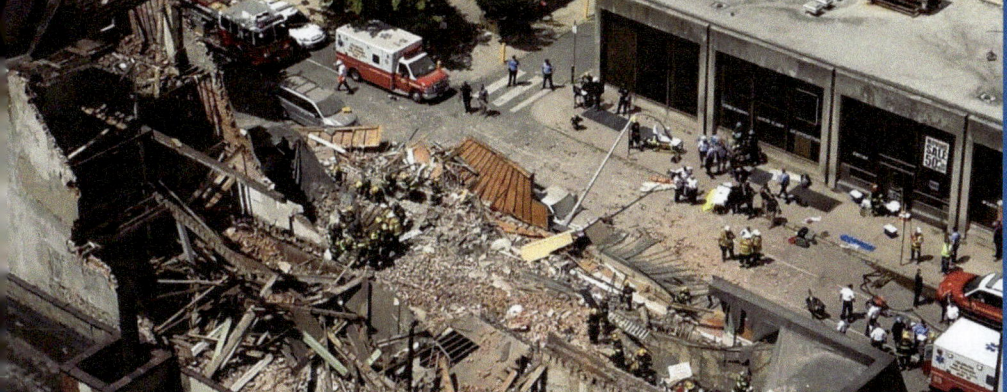

Explosions and Blast Injuries

LESSON OBJECTIVES

At the completion of this lesson, you should be able to do the following:

· State the triage and PPE considerations in disasters involving explosions.

· List the common injury patterns with explosions.

· Explain the management considerations in blast injuries and multisystem trauma.

General Considerations

An EMS practitioner is much more likely to encounter injury from conventional explosives than a chemical, biologic, or nuclear attack. This chapter covers the many causes of explosions, intentional blasts, closed- versus open-space explosions, the imperative of situational awareness, and the EMS interface with law enforcement. It also reviews triage considerations, personal protective equipment (PPE) for EMS practitioners, transport considerations, and special populations in the context of explosions.

The Many Causes of Explosions

Not only can explosions occur in homes (primarily due to gas leaks, propane grills, fires, or residential chemicals), but they are also an occupational hazard in many industries (e.g., mining, demolition, chemical manufacturing, handling of fuel or dust-producing substances such as grain). Industrial explosions result from chemical spills, fires, equipment malfunction, or electrical/machinery malfunctions, and they may produce fires, toxic fumes, building collapse, secondary explosions, falling debris, and large numbers of casualties. Other common causes of explosions are the rupture of pressurized containment

vessels, such as a boiler; motor vehicle collisions; and split-rim tire ruptures. In addition, intentional blasts may occur for various reasons, including assault, arson, and terrorism. Terrorists worldwide are increasingly using bombs, especially improvised explosive devices (IEDs), against civilian targets. These inexpensive devices are made from easily obtained materials and produce devastating and chaotic results.

Closed- vs. Open-Space Explosions

Closed-space explosions are associated with greater mortality and morbidity than open-space explosions due to the reflection of the blast wave back onto the victims rather than the dispersal of the blast wave into the surrounding area and associated structural collapse. Primary blast injury was noted in 38% of the survivors of a closed-space explosion in Jerusalem compared to 0.6% of the survivors of an open-space explosion in Beirut. This pattern was also seen in the three bombs detonated in the London subway system in 2005. Two of the three bombs exploded in wide tunnels, resulting in 6 and 7 fatalities, respectively. The third device detonated in a narrow tunnel, causing 26 fatalities.

The Imperative of Situational Awareness

Detonations expose EMS practitioners to many risks. As such, maintaining situational awareness is crucial. Along with situational awareness comes the need for accountability of all personnel on the scene, including clear communications and plans for responder evacuation.

In the case of an explosive detonation, there may be fire, spilled hazardous materials, power-line hazards, and risk of falling debris or subsidence (the creation of craters) (**Figure 8-1**). One emergency responder was killed by falling debris in response to the Oklahoma City bombing in 1995. When the buildings collapsed in the 2001 World Trade Center attack, many emergency responders were killed, including 343 firefighters, 15 emergency medical technicians (EMTs), and 3 law enforcement officers.

A further risk is the possibility of **secondary devices**. A second bomb could be placed at the scene of the incident, set to explode after the arrival of emergency responders, with the intention of increasing injury, confusion, and panic. EMS practitioners must adjust and adapt their response based on the evolving situation and focus on prompt extraction to a cold zone.

Law Enforcement Interface

An explosive event scene may be a crime scene, so preserving evidence is very important; however, it does not take precedence over saving lives (**Figure 8-2**). EMS practitioners should, therefore, be guided by principles of criminal investigation and evidence preservation. EMS practitioners should make an extra effort to be aware of crime scene indicators, evidence preservation, and chain of custody. They should avoid disturbing or compromising evidence. EMS practitioners should also be aware of possible suspects or perpetrators.

Triage Considerations

Accurate and efficient triage is extremely important, and overtriage can delay recognition and treatment of patients with hidden or delayed injuries. Most triage systems start with an attempt to direct those who are ambulatory (the walking wounded) to a safe area and to determine if patients can follow commands. However, after an explosion, temporary hearing loss will affect most patients' ability to respond to verbal commands. EMS practitioners must be prepared for how hearing loss will impact triage. Visual sign boards and written communication might be needed. Primary triage should focus on identifying and rapidly temporizing life threats: massive hemorrhage, airway compromise, and tension pneumothorax.

Triage for an explosive event poses other unique challenges, as the blast wave can cause severe internal injuries that are not immediately apparent, which is dangerous for patients. These patients may also have combined blast, ballistic, and burn injuries, including subtle-appearing soft-tissue injuries that can be difficult to detect. Terrorist bombs often contain nails, bolts, and other sharp objects that produce unique injury patterns. Bombs or explosive devices are often detonated in enclosed spaces such as buses or buildings, increasing the effects of the pressure wave. Patients may present with internal injuries out of proportion with their external appearance; in other words, they may initially appear fine but quickly develop shock from internal injuries. During secondary triage, EMS practitioners must be prepared to reassess for signs of internal injury and remain vigilant for signs of blast injuries.

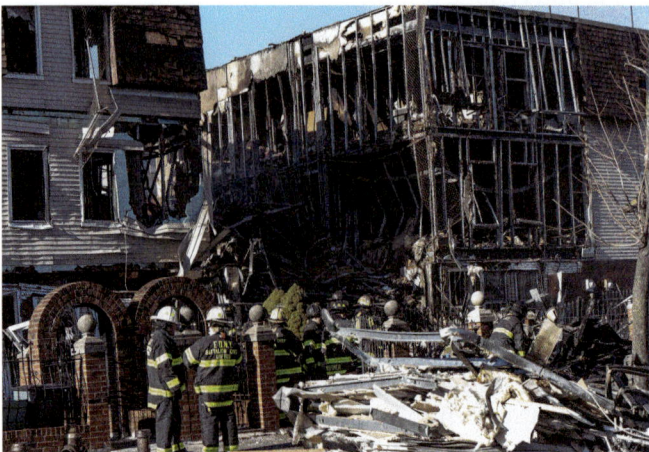

Figure 8-1 Explosions can produce numerous hazards, including fire, spilled hazardous materials, downed power-line hazards, and falling debris or subsidence (the creation of craters).
© Lev Radin/Sipa USA/AP Photo

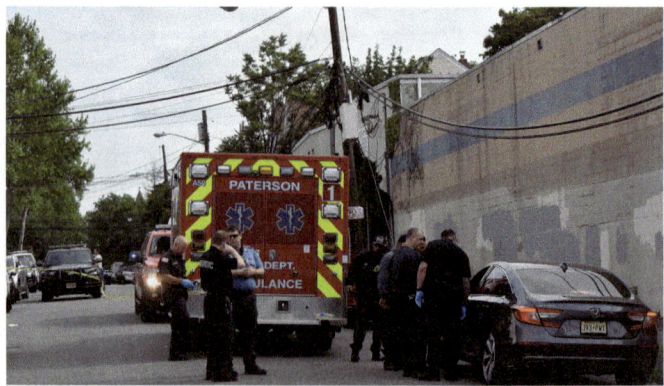

Figure 8-2 The EMS practitioner's role may sometimes involve consideration of law enforcement's needs.
© Kyle Mazza/SOPA Images/Shutterstock

Terrorist bombing events usually result in predominantly noncritical injuries to patients. Studies report that around 20% of casualties of a terrorist bombing have critical injuries. Medical resources may be overwhelmed if they face hundreds of noncritical patients who do not need immediate attention. This overtriage (which may be self-triage) can delay the recognition and treatment of patients with urgent and treatable life-threatening injuries.

Transport Considerations

Patients requiring transport must be brought to an appropriate medical treatment facility, such as designated trauma and burn centers, for further evaluation and management. Patient arrival at hospitals is usually bimodal, with ambulatory patients arriving first and more critically ill patients arriving later by ambulance. EMS practitioners should consider the volume of patients arriving at the nearest hospitals when determining the destination of patients transported by ambulance from the blast scene. In blast events where many of the hospitals closest to the explosion have sustained substantial damage, the distribution patterns have been much more complex and harder to predict.

For instance, during the 2020 Beirut Port ammonium nitrate explosion, three hospitals closest to the port sustained enough structural damage that they could not receive blast victims and had to transfer patients and injured staff to other facilities. Other hospitals (those within a 3-mile [5-km] radius) were so overwhelmed with patients in the 54 hours following the blast that some documented only those patients admitted to the operating room or intensive care unit. Patients who received minor care (e.g., wound sutures or stapling) were unregistered casualties, creating a significant undercount of those affected by the explosion. Before initiating transport, EMS practitioners should check if the nearby hospitals have sustained damage and can take patients.

Special Populations

In patients who are pregnant, especially those in their second or third trimester, placental injuries and maternal–fetal hemorrhage are possible. These patients should be transported to a hospital with labor and delivery capabilities.

Assessment of pediatric patients is complex. Pulmonary contusions are common in this patient population. Therefore, EMS personnel should consider transporting these patients to a pediatric specialty center.

Geriatric patients generally have underlying medical conditions that may be exacerbated. It is also critical to remember that older adults are more prone to orthopedic injuries and that any chest trauma can cause serious pulmonary problems.

When interacting with patients with disabilities, EMS practitioners should consider underlying conditions.

Explosives
Categories of Explosives

Explosives are categorized as **high-order explosives (HE)** or **low-order explosives (LE)**. High- and low-order explosives cause different injury patterns due to the presence or absence of the overpressurization wave. Practically speaking, it may be difficult for the initial EMS practitioners to differentiate between a high- versus low-order explosion immediately following a blast unless the explosive agent is known. The focus should always be on scene safety, initial triage, and treatment of life-threatening injuries.

High-order explosives react almost instantaneously and produce a defining supersonic overpressurization shock wave (**Figure 8-3**). Examples include TNT, C-4, Semtex, nitroglycerin, dynamite, ammonium nitrate–fuel oil (ANFO), and gelignite. These agents are associated with primary blast injuries because they produce a supersonic shock wave or **overpressure phenomenon**. High-order explosives have a sharp, shattering effect (*brisance*) that can pulverize bone and soft tissue, create blast overpressure injuries (**barotrauma**) from the rapid expansion of gas in the body, and propel debris at ballistic speeds (*fragmentation*), causing penetrating trauma. Note that a high-order explosive may result in a low-order explosion, particularly if the explosive has deteriorated because of age (e.g., plastic explosive Semtex) or, in some cases, has become wet (dynamite). The reverse, however, is not true; a low-order explosive cannot produce a high-order explosion.

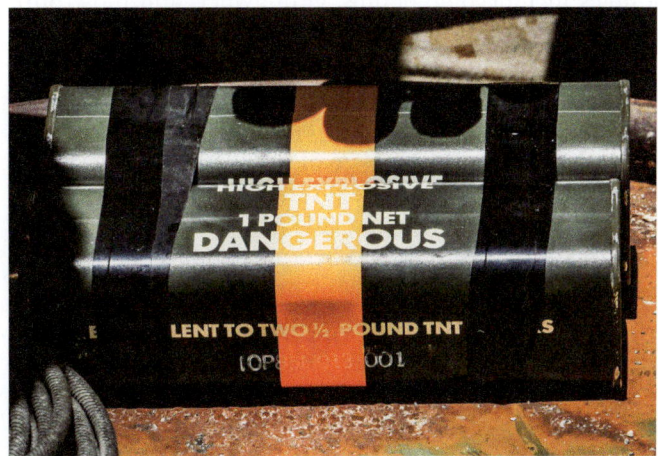

Figure 8-3 TNT is an example of a high-order explosive.
Courtesy of the U.S. Department of Defense.

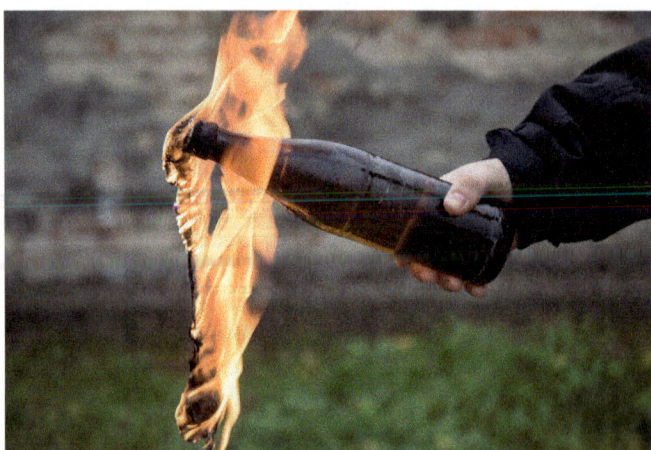

Figure 8-4 A Molotov cocktail is an example of a low-order explosive.

© SasaStock/Shutterstock

Low-order explosives create a subsonic explosion and lack an overpressurization wave (**Figure 8-4**). Examples include pipe bombs, gunpowder, and most pure petroleum-based bombs (e.g., Molotov cocktails, aircraft improvised as guided missiles). Explosions resulting from container rupture and ignition of volatile compounds fall into this category. The type and amount of low-order explosive determine the size of the blast associated with device detonation. This makes the approach to the scene and the location for staging EMS practitioners and equipment critical decisions. When responding to a scene involving a suspicious device or a potential secondary device, all EMS practitioners must stage at a safe distance from the site in case of a second detonation.

Explosion Terminology

A **blast wave** results from the sudden conversion of a high-order explosive from a solid (or liquid) to a gas. This wave dissipates rapidly over time and distance. The leading edge of a blast wave is the **shock wave**, which travels at supersonic speeds and carries energy that strikes and passes through objects in its path, causing damage. After the detonation of a high-order explosive, the force of the explosion pushes all the air out of the area immediately around the detonation site, creating a sudden vacuum. Once the force of the explosion has been spent, all the air that was pushed out rushes back in response to the vacuum. The result is a powerful **blast wind** that can cause objects and debris to be sucked back in toward the explosion site.

Mechanisms of Injury

Types of Blast Injuries

Traumatic injuries caused by explosions are generally divided into primary, secondary, and tertiary blast injuries. In addition to the injuries that result directly from the blast, additional categories of injuries classified as quaternary and quinary effects result from complications or toxic effects related to the explosive or contaminants. These injuries may occur in combination in victims of explosions. Injuries from bombings or explosions affect the air-containing organs more substantially than other organs.

Primary blast injuries result from detonation of high-order explosives and the consequent interaction of the blast overpressure wave with the body or tissue producing stress and **shear waves**. A victim may suffer primary blast injury depending on the victim's proximity to the explosion and shielding from or augmentation of the shock wave if the explosion occurs in a closed space. Primary blast injury occurs in gas-filled organs such as the lung, bowel, and middle ear. The injury to the tissue

Common Injury Patterns Associated with Explosions

Primary blast injuries:

- Blast lung: pulmonary barotraumas
- Head: traumatic brain injury, concussion
- Ear: tympanic membrane (eardrum) rupture and middle ear damage
- Abdomen: hemorrhage and organ perforation

Secondary blast injuries:

- Trauma to the head, neck, chest, abdomen, and extremities in the form of penetrating and blunt trauma
- Fractures
- Traumatic amputations
- Soft-tissue injuries

Tertiary blast injuries:

- Head injuries
- Skull fractures
- Bone fractures
- Blunt and/or penetrating thoracoabdominal trauma

Quaternary blast injuries:

- Burns
- Head injuries
- Asthma, chronic obstructive pulmonary disease (COPD)
- Other breathing problems
- Acute coronary syndromes
- Hyperglycemia
- Hypertension
- Crush injuries

Modified from Centers for disease control & prevention & U.S Department of Health & human services, American College of Emergency Physicians. Bombings: injury patterns and care: blast injuries seminar curriculum guide. Accessed May 31, 2023. https://www.acep.org/imports/clinical-and-practice-management/resources/ems-and-disaster-preparedness/disaster-preparedness-grant-projects/bombings-injury-patterns-and-care/

occurs at the gas–fluid interface, causing the violent collapse of that organ, followed by an equally rapid and violent expansion, resulting in tissue injury.

Secondary blast injuries are caused by flying debris and bomb fragments and debris carried by the blast wind, resulting in penetrating and blunt trauma. These projectiles may be components of the bomb itself, as in military weapons designed to fragment, or they may be parts of improvised bombs augmented with nails, screws, and bolts. Secondary blast injuries are the most common cause of death in a blast event.

Tertiary blast injuries are caused by the blast wind throwing the victim's body, resulting in tumbling and collisions with other objects. This can result in the whole spectrum of injuries associated with blunt trauma and even penetrating trauma such as impalement.

Following the blast itself, **quaternary effects** may be seen. These injuries include burns and toxicities from fuel and metals, trauma from structural collapse, and septic syndromes from soil and environmental contamination of wounds.

The increasing threat of radiation-, chemical-, or biologic-enhanced explosives (i.e., dirty bombs) has given rise to a fifth category of effects called **quinary effects**, which includes injuries caused by radiation, chemicals, or biologic agents and projectiles such as bone fragments of a suicide bomber.

EMS practitioners will be confronted with penetrating, blunt, and thermal injuries and possibly survivors with primary blast injuries. Practically speaking, secondary and tertiary blast injuries often result in immediate life-threatening conditions such as severe hemorrhage and are the most common cause of death. Treatment for most secondary, tertiary, and quaternary injuries follows established protocols for that specific injury.

Blast Lung Injury (BLI)

Blast lung injury (BLI) is a major cause of morbidity and mortality among blast victims both at the scene and at the hospital among initial survivors (**Figure 8-5**). The impact of the blast wave results in tearing, hemorrhage, and edema of lung tissue. Examination of the lungs shows ecchymoses, petechiae, lacerations, and increased weight due to edema and hemorrhage. Damage also occurs to the airway epithelium and intra-alveolar septa. These pathologic changes result in ventilation–perfusion mismatch and the potential for air embolism.

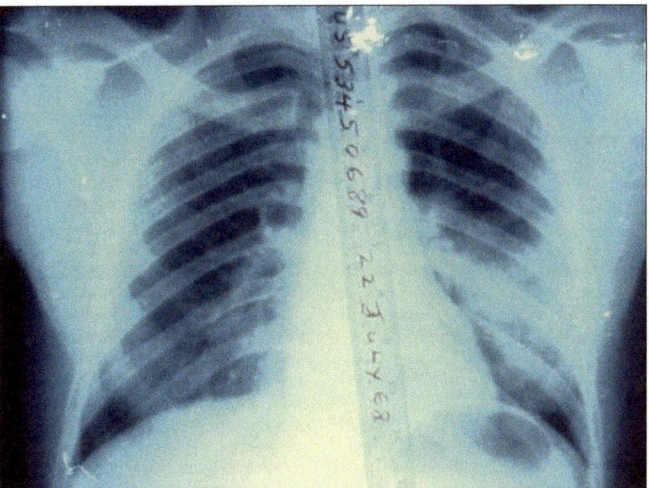

Figure 8-5 Radiograph of a blast lung injury.
© Rapp Halour/Alamy Stock Photo

Blast Lung Injury: What Prehospital Care Practitioners Need to Know

Few civilian prehospital care practitioners in the United States have experience treating patients with explosion-related injuries. BLI presents unique triage, diagnostic, and management challenges and directly results from the blast wave from high-order explosive detonations upon the body. Persons in enclosed-space explosions or those close to the explosion are at a higher risk. BLI is a clinical diagnosis characterized by respiratory difficulty and hypoxia. It can occur, although rarely, without obvious external injury to the chest. It is often not an immediate manifestation but develops over several hours during the overall course of resuscitation.

Clinical Presentation

- Symptoms may include dyspnea, hemoptysis, cough, and chest pain.

- Signs may include tachypnea, hypoxia, cyanosis, apnea, wheezing, decreased breath sounds, and hemodynamic instability.

- Victims with greater than 10% body surface area burns, skull fractures, and penetrating torso or head injuries may be more likely to have BLI.

- Hemothorax or pneumothorax may occur.

- Due to the tearing of the pulmonary and vascular tree, air may enter the arterial circulation (*air emboli*) and result in embolic events involving the central nervous system, retinal arteries, or coronary arteries, resulting in stroke-like symptoms.

- Clinical evidence of BLI may be present during initial evaluation; however, it more typically presents several hours after the initial injury during resuscitation and has been reported to occur as late as 24 to 48 hours after an explosion.

- Other injuries may also often be present.

Prehospital Management Considerations

Although scene safety is always a major consideration for prehospital care practitioners, incidents such as these often require emergency responders of all types to enter the scene before the scene can be declared completely secure. Practitioners must remain aware of their surroundings, be observant of possible additional devices, and consider other hazards that may have resulted from the primary explosion. Patient assessment and management steps are as follows, assuming direct and indirect threat potential has been mitigated, and practitioners have a safe operating environment:

- Initial triage, trauma resuscitation, and transport of patients should follow standard protocols for multiple injured patients or mass casualties, including assessment and treatment following the XABCDE primary survey or MARCH algorithm (control **M**assive hemorrhage, **A**irway, **R**espiration, **C**irculation, and **H**ead and **H**ypothermia).

- Note the patient's location and the surrounding environment. Explosions in a confined space result in a higher incidence of primary blast injury, including lung injury.

- All patients with suspected or confirmed BLI should receive supplemental high-flow oxygen sufficient to prevent hypoxemia.

- Impending airway compromise requires immediate intervention.

- If ventilatory failure is imminent or occurs, patients should be intubated, however, prehospital care practitioners must realize that mechanical ventilation and positive pressure may increase the risk of alveolar rupture, pneumothorax, and air embolism in BLI patients.

- High-flow oxygen should be administered if air embolism is suspected, and the patient should be placed in a semi–left lateral or left lateral position.

- Clinical evidence of or suspicion of a hemothorax or pneumothorax warrants close observation. Chest decompression should be performed for patients clinically presenting with a tension pneumothorax. Close observation is warranted for any patient with suspicion of a BLI transported by air, as even small changes in altitude can exacerbate barotrauma.

- Fluids should be administered judiciously, as overzealous fluid administration in the patient with BLI may result in volume overload and worsening pulmonary status.

- Patients with BLI should be transported rapidly to the nearest appropriate facility in accordance with community response plans for mass-casualty events.

Data from Centers for Disease Control and Prevention, National Center for Injury Prevention and Control, Division of Injury Response. Blast injuries: fact sheets for professionals. Published March 1, 2012. Accessed January 26, 2022. https://stacks.cdc.gov/view/cdc/21571.

Clinical manifestations of BLI include tachypnea, hypoxia, cyanosis, apnea, wheezing, decreased breath sounds, hemoptysis, cough, chest pain, dyspnea, and hemodynamic instability. Symptoms are usually present at the time of evaluation but can also have an onset several hours after the explosion. Among survivors of primary blast injury, clinical manifestations may be present immediately or may have a delayed onset of 24 to 48 hours.

Since primary blast injuries are often not immediately apparent, care at the scene should include monitoring for frothy secretions and respiratory distress, sequential oxygen saturation (SpO_2) measurements, and provision of oxygen. Decreased SpO_2 is a red flag for early BLI even before symptoms begin. Fluid administration must be carefully managed, with care taken to avoid fluid overload. Patients with any complaints or findings suspicious of pulmonary (or abdominal) blast injury should be transported to the hospital, as they are at significant risk for clinical deterioration.

Tympanic Membrane Rupture

Patients who arrive at a medical facility from an explosive event should be evaluated and resuscitated per standard trauma protocols. All patients should have a secondary evaluation and examination to identify all blast-related injuries, including perforated tympanic membranes. Tympanic membrane rupture may result from exposure to the blast overpressurization wave (**Figure 8-6**). It may be found in victims with severe pulmonary, intestinal, or other injuries, or it may be found in isolation. The presence of tympanic membrane rupture does not necessarily indicate that more sinister blast injuries exist. Likewise, its absence does not exclude the possibility of more serious injuries. Other ear injuries, besides tympanic membrane rupture, such as ossicular disruption, cochlear damage, and foreign bodies, are also possible. Treatment is supportive, and a detailed secondary assessment should be performed to evaluate for other injuries.

Abdominal Injuries (Blast Abdomen)

Abdominal injuries (also called blast abdomen) include abdominal hemorrhage and abdominal organ perforation. They may initially be missed in unconscious patients. Organ perforation may have a delayed presentation because infection and inflammation take time to develop. Clinical manifestations of abdominal injuries include abdominal tenderness or testicular pain, tenesmus (the feeling of having to defecate), rectal bleeding, solid organ lacerations, rebound tenderness, guarding, absent bowel sounds, signs of shock/hypovolemia, nausea, and vomiting.

Head Injuries

Primary blast waves can cause concussions or mild traumatic brain injury without a direct blow to the head (**Figure 8-7**). EMS practitioners should consider the

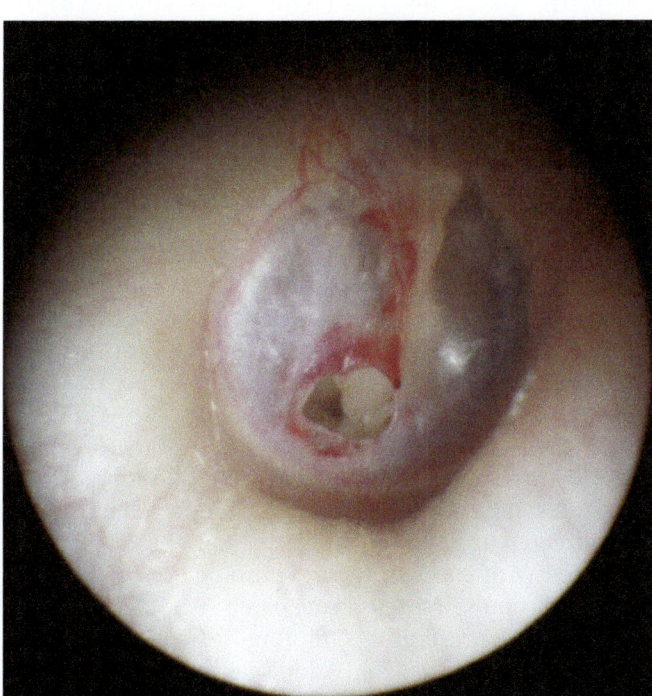

Figure 8-6 Posttraumatic perforation of the tympanic membrane.
© Mikhail V. Komarov/Shutterstock

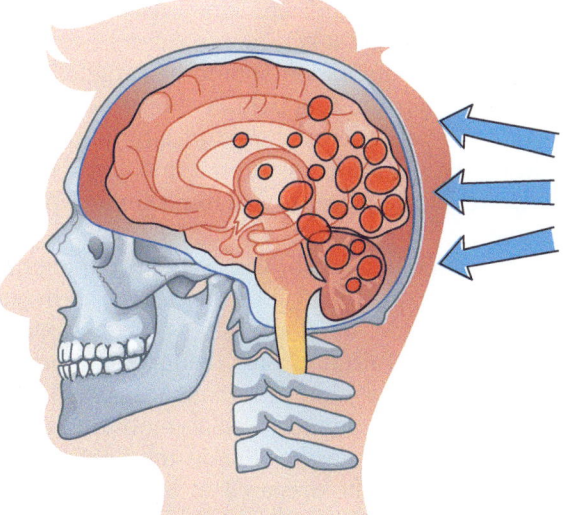

Figure 8-7 Primary blast waves can cause concussions or mild traumatic brain injury without a direct blow to the head.
© VectorMine/Shutterstock

victim's proximity to the blast, particularly if the patient reports loss of consciousness, headache, confusion, fatigue, poor concentration, lethargy, amnesia, lightheadedness, or other constitutional symptoms. The symptoms of concussion and posttraumatic stress disorder can be similar.

Multisystem Trauma

The likelihood of multisystem trauma is increased in blast victims. The management principles for these patients are similar to those for trauma from other mechanisms. As nuances of the environment of injury can greatly affect the relative predominance of primary versus secondary and higher-order injuries, patients may present with internal injuries out of proportion with their external appearance. For example, a patient closer to the blast but shielded by a concrete wall may have significant internal injuries from primary blast effects but appear less severely injured on initial examination than a patient located farther away from the explosion with secondary blast injuries from flying debris resulting in many superficial lacerations. Practitioners should closely monitor all casualties, reassess vital signs frequently, and retriage to higher categories as needed.

Combined injuries, especially blast and burn or blast and crush injuries, are common during an explosive event. It is important to avoid tunnel vision that would address one injury but not another and thus cause harm. In all cases of combined injury, control of life-threatening hemorrhage, airway management, and oxygenation/ventilation are critical to survival and should be achieved with standard techniques.

In a combined burn/blast injury, although the burn injury will require significant amounts of fluid resuscitation, care must be taken to avoid fluid overload. In the field, fluid resuscitation should be targeted to vital signs to avoid hypotension; boluses should be given only as needed. These patients should ideally be brought to a facility with expertise in trauma and burn management; however, transport to a trauma center should be prioritized.

With a combined crush/blast injury, the patient will need IV fluid boluses to reduce the danger of hyperkalemic cardiac arrest upon releasing the entrapped tissue. A standard 20-mL/kg bolus (about 2 L in an adult) and an infusion of sodium bicarbonate may offer some protection. Still, continuous cardiac monitoring should be established as soon as possible in the field, and EMS practitioners should be prepared to treat hyperkalemia pharmacologically (with calcium/albuterol).

Crush Injuries

Crush injury occurs when prolonged force or pressure is applied to a body part. In disasters, the lower extremities, upper extremities, and trunk are most likely to sustain crush injuries. Approximately 3% to 20% of the survivors of earthquakes have sustained a crush injury, and approximately 40% of survivors from collapsed buildings will have crush injuries. Crush syndrome refers to a combination of physiologic events. The trauma of a crush injury to muscle causes release of both myoglobin and potassium. Once the patient has been extricated, the affected limb suddenly becomes reperfused with new blood; at the same time, the old blood with elevated levels of myoglobin and potassium is washed out of the injured area and into the rest of the body. Elevated potassium can result in life-threatening cardiac dysrhythmias, and free myoglobin will produce tea- or cola-colored urine and will eventually result in renal failure. It is the combination of these events that is typically described as crush syndrome.

The greatest initial danger for crush injury is after the crushed limb is released. It is important to initiate fluid resuscitation for the patient with severe or prolonged entrapment of a limb (more than a hand or foot) before the crushed tissue is released. In certain contexts, alkalinization of the urine may be performed by administering a sodium bicarbonate infusion (per local protocols). Practitioners should be prepared for sudden hemodynamic instability, arrhythmia, and mental status changes as the patient is extricated. They should also be ready to treat for hyperkalemia.

Compartment Syndrome

Compartment syndrome refers to a limb-threatening condition in which the blood supply to an extremity is compromised by increased pressure within that limb. The two most common causes of compartment syndrome are hemorrhage within a compartment from a fracture or vascular injury and third-space edema that forms when ischemic muscle tissue is reperfused after a period of diminished or absent blood flow. It may occur in settings similar to crush injury as well as due to fractures, penetrating trauma, and prolonged immobilization. Compartment syndrome can lead to crush injury/syndrome if left untreated or if inadequately treated. The "5 Ps" often associated with compartment syndrome are pain, pallor, paresthesia, pulselessness, and paralysis. Severe pain is often the first presenting symptom; loss of pulses often does not occur until late. Additionally, numbness, tingling, or pain may be present in the entire lower leg and foot. Prehospital care includes analgesia and immobilization but does *not* include use of constricting bandages or tourniquets (unless life-threatening external bleeding is present). EMS practitioners should assess for and treat other injuries. Compartment syndrome is a surgical emergency that requires rapid transport.

Incendiary Agents

Incendiary agents are typically encountered in the military and are used to burn equipment, vehicles, and structures. Terrorists may use them to increase the lethality of improvised explosive devices. The three incendiary agents most often recognized are thermite, magnesium, and white phosphorus. All three are highly flammable compounds that burn at extremely high temperatures.

Thermite

Thermite is powdered aluminum and iron oxide that burns furiously at 3,600°F (1,982°C) and scatters molten iron. Its primary mechanism of injury is partial-thickness or full-thickness burns. Primary survey and secondary assessment are performed with interventions directed at treating burns. Thermite wounds can be irrigated with copious amounts of water, and any residual particles or material is subsequently removed.

Magnesium

Magnesium is a powdered or solid metal that burns furiously hot. In addition to its ability to cause partial-thickness or full-thickness burns, magnesium can react with tissue fluid and cause alkali burns. The same chemical reaction produces hydrogen gas, which can cause the wound to bubble or can result in subcutaneous emphysema. Inhalation of magnesium dust can produce respiratory symptoms, including cough, tachypnea, hypoxia, wheezing, pneumonitis, and airway burns. Residual magnesium particles in a wound will react with water, so irrigation is discouraged until the wounds can be debrided and the particulates removed. If irrigation is required for other reasons, such as decontamination of another suspected material, care should be taken to ensure flushing or removal of magnesium particles from the wound.

White Phosphorus

White phosphorus is a solid that spontaneously ignites when exposed to air, causing a yellow flame and white smoke. When it comes in contact with skin, it can quickly result in partial- or full-thickness burns. It can become embedded in the skin, propelled by the blast of munitions. The substance will continue to burn in the skin if exposed to air. Its systemic absorption can lead to lethal heart, liver, and kidney injury.

EMS practitioners can decrease the likelihood of combustion in the skin by immersing the affected areas in water or applying saline-soaked dressings. Oily or greasy dressings are avoided; because white phosphorus is lipid soluble, application of these dressings may increase the likelihood of systemic absorption and toxicity. Contaminated clothing should be removed, as it may catch fire if the white phosphorus reignites. White phosphorus fluoresces under ultraviolet light, which can be used to ensure thorough decontamination.

SUMMARY

- Traumatic injuries caused by explosions are divided into the following categories: primary blast injury, secondary blast injury, tertiary blast injury, and quaternary/quinary effects. These injuries may occur in combination in victims of explosions.
- Common injuries seen in blasts are musculoskeletal injuries, blast lung injury, blast-induced brain and eye trauma, and tympanic membrane rupture.
- Hearing loss impacts the methods used to triage explosion victims.
- In primary blast injuries, monitor for signs of blast lung, including frothy secretions, respiratory distress, and sequential (serial) oxygen saturation. Provide oxygen and fluid administration to vital sign goals.
- Due to the likelihood of multisystem trauma in bomb victims, closely monitor all casualties, reassess vital signs frequently, and retriage to higher categories as needed.
- Patients may present with internal injuries out of proportion with their external appearance.
- Before transporting patients to nearby hospitals, check if the nearby hospitals have sustained damage and can take patients.

References and Additional Resources

Almogy G, Mintz Y, Zamir G, et al. Suicide bombing attacks: can external signs predict internal injuries? *Ann Surg.* 2006;243(4):541–546.

American College of Emergency Physicians. *Bombings: Injury Patterns and Care.* https://www.acep.org/imports/clinical-and-practice-management/resources/ems-and-disaster-preparedness/disaster-preparedness-grant-projects/bombings-injury-patterns-and-care/. Accessed May 31, 2023.

Armed Forces Radiobiology Research Institute (AFRRI). *Medical Management of Radiological Casualties.* AFRRI; 2003.

Arnold J, Halpern P, Tsai M. Mass casualty terrorist bombings: a comparison of outcomes by bombing type. *Ann Emerg Med.* 2004;43:263–273.

Arnold JL, Tsai MC, Halpern P, et al. Mass-casualty, terrorist bombings: epidemiological outcomes, resource utilization, and time course of emergency needs (Part I). *Prehosp Disaster Med.* 2003;18(3):220–234.

Avidan V, Hersch M, Armon Y, et al. Blast lung injury: clinical manifestations, treatment, and outcome. *Am J Surg.* 2005;190(6):927–931.

Branica S, Dawidowsky K, Kovač-Bilić L, Bilić M. Silicon foil patching for blast tympanic membrane perforation: a retrospective study. *Croatian Med J.* 2019;60(6):503

Caseby NG, Porter MF. Blast injury to the lungs: clinical presentation, management and course. *Injury.* 1976;8:1 12.

Centers for Disease Control and Prevention. Explosions and blast injuries: a primer for clinicians. Updated May 9, 2003. https://www.cdc.gov/masstrauma/preparedness/primer.pdf. Accessed January 31, 2022.

Cohn SM. Pulmonary contusion: review of the clinical entity. *J Trauma.* 1997;42:973–979.

Collins AJ, Burzstein S. Renal failure in disasters. *Crit Care Clin.* 1991;7:421.

Coppel DL. Blast injuries of the lungs. *Br J Surg.* 1976;63:735–737.

DePalma RG, Burris DG, Champion HR, et al. Blast injuries. *N Engl J Med.* 2005;352(13):1335–1342.

Edwards DS, Mcmenemy L, Stapley SA, Patel HD, Clasper JC. 40 years of terrorist bombings: a meta-analysis of the casualty and injury profile. *Injury.* 2016;47(3):646–652.

Frykberg ER, Tepas JJ, Alexander RH. The 1983 Beirut Airport terrorist bombing: injury patterns and implications for disaster management. *Am Surg.* 1989;55:134–141.

Garner MJ, Brett SJ. Mechanisms of injury by explosive devices. *Anesthesiol Clin.* 2007;25(1):147–160.

Halpern P, Tsai MC, Arnold JL, et al. Mass-casualty, terrorist bombings: implications for emergency department and hospital emergency response (Part II). *Prehosp Disaster Med.* 2003;18(3):235–241.

Irizarry L. White phosphorus exposure. Medscape. Updated January 6, 2022. http://emedicine.medscape.com/article/833585-overview. Accessed January 31, 2022.

Kapur GB, Hutson HR, Davis MA, Rice PL. The United States twenty-year experience with bombing incidents: implications for terrorism preparedness and medical response. *J Trauma.* 2005;59:1436–1444.

Katz E, Ofek B, Adler J, et al. Primary blast injury after a bomb explosion in a civilian bus. *Ann Surg.* 1989;209:484–488.

Kluger Y, Nimrod A, Biderman P, et al. Case report: the quinary pattern of blast injury. *J Emerg Mgmt.* 2006;4(1):51–55.

Leibovici D, Gofrit ON, Shapira SC. Eardrum perforation in explosion survivors: is it a marker of pulmonary blast injury? *Ann Emerg Med.* 1999;34:168–172.

Mallonee S, Shariat S, Stennies G, et al. Physical injuries and fatalities resulting from the Oklahoma City bombing. *JAMA.* 1996;276:382–787.

Mansour HA, Bitar E, Fares Y, Makdessi AA, et al. The Beirut Port explosion: injury trends from a mass survey of emergency admissions. *Lancet.* 2021;398:21–22.

Melnikova N, Orr MF, Wu J, Christensen B. Injuries from methamphetamine-related chemical incidents—five states, 2001–2012. *Morb Mortal Wkly Rep.* 2015;64(33):909–912.

Michaelson M, Taitelman U, Bshouty Z, et al. Crush syndrome: experience from the Lebanon war, 1982. *Isr J Med Sci.* 1984;20:305.

National Association of Emergency Medical Technicians. *Advanced Medical Life Support.* 3rd ed. Jones & Bartlett Learning; 2021.

National Association of Emergency Medical Technicians. *Prehospital Trauma Life Support.* 10th ed. Jones & Bartlett Learning; 2023.

National Center for Injury Prevention and Control, Division of Injury Response; Centers for Disease Control and Prevention. Blast injuries: fact sheets for professionals. Published March 1, 2012. https://stacks.cdc.gov/view/cdc/21571. Accessed June 13, 2023.

Nelson TJ, Wall DB, Stedje-Larsen ET, et al. Predictors of mortality in close proximity blast injuries during Operation Iraqi Freedom. *J Am Coll Surg.* 2006;202(3):418–422.

Peleg K, Limor A, Stein M, et al. Gunshot and explosion injuries: characteristics, outcomes, and implications for care of terror-related injuries in Israel. *Ann Surg.* 2004;239(3):311–318.

Pierce B. How rare are large, multiple-fatality work-related incidents? *Accid Anal Prev.* 2016;96:88–100.

Plurad DS. Blast injury. *Mil Med.* 2011 Mar;176(3):276–282.

Pretto EA, Angus D, Abrams J, et al. An analysis of prehospital mortality in an earthquake. *Prehosp Disaster Med.* 1994;9:107.

Sever MS, Vanholder R, Lameire N. Management of crush-related injuries after disasters. *N Engl J Med.* 2006;354:1052.

Sinnott JD, Johnston A, Pemberton P. Blast lung. *BMJ.* 2015;350:h363.

Sorkine P, Nimrod A, Biderman P, et al. The quinary (Vth) injury pattern of blast (Abstract). *J Trauma.* 2007;56(1):232.

Tappan J. Magnesium and thermite poisoning. *Medscape.* Updated June 28, 2023. http://emedicine.medscape.com/article/833495-overview. Accessed July 21, 2023.

U.S. Bomb Data Center. *Explosive Incidents 2007: 2007 USBDC Explosives Statistics.* U.S. Bomb Data Center; 2007.

U.S. Bomb Data Center. *Explosives Incident Report (EIR)—2019.* Redstone Arsenal, AL: U.S. Bomb Data Center; 2019. https://www.atf.gov/file/143481/download. Accessed May 31, 2023.

Wightman JM, Gladish JL. Explosions and blast injuries. *Ann Emerg Med.* 2001;37:664–678.

GLOSSARY

Active shooter An individual actively engaged in killing or attempting to kill people in a confined space or other populated area.

Acute radiation syndrome A serious illness that can result from exposure to very high levels of radiation, usually over a short period. The amount of radiation that a person's body absorbs is called the radiation dose.

Aerosol precautions Infectious disease transmission through very small droplets expelled from an infected respiratory tract.

Airborne transmission Precautions recommended to reduce the likelihood of transmission of microorganisms by the airborne route.

Air-purifying respirator (APR) A device that uses a filter, canister, or cartridge to remove contaminants from ambient air that passes through the air-purifying component and makes the air safe to breathe.

Ambulance strike team An ICS resource consisting of five ambulances and a supervisor or support vehicle operating under a shared communication system.

Barotrauma Injury to air-containing organs that results from a change in air pressure.

Biologic agent A bacterium, virus, or toxin that can be used as a weapon of mass destruction.

Bioterrorism When biologic agents are used on the human population, animals, and crops to cause harm or invoke fear.

Blast lung injury (BLI) Results from exposure to high-order explosive blast overpressure wave; lung damage varies from scattered petechiae to contusions and pulmonary hemorrhage.

Blast wave A sharply defined wave front of increased pressure that propagates outward from the center of an explosion.

Blast wind The result of the sudden displacement of air from an explosion.

Blister agents A chemical that creates burnlike injuries; used as a weapon of mass destruction.

Casualty collection point A location used for the collection, triage, treatment, and evacuation of casualties from a multiple-casualty incident.

Category A bioterrorism agents Bioterrorism agents that pose the highest risk to national security and public health.

Category B bioterrorism agents Bioterrorism agents that are moderately easy to disseminate, result in moderate morbidity and low mortality rates, and require specific enhancements of the CDC's diagnostic capacity and disease surveillance—water safety threats, food safety threats, toxins, and alphaviruses.

Category C bioterrorism agents Emerging pathogens that pose a risk due to the potential to be engineered for mass dissemination, availability, ease of production and dissemination, high morbidity and mortality rates, and potential for major health impact.

CBRNE Abbreviation for the constellation of chemical, biologic, radiologic, nuclear, and explosive hazards.

Chemical placard A diamond-shaped sign that is color coded to identify the hazardous agent as being flammable, combustible, poisonous, radioactive, gaseous, explosive, oxidizing, infectious, or corrosive.

Cold zone Also called the **green zone**, evacuation zone, or patient care zone, it is the area outside the hot and warm zones that is not contaminated (or with radiation < 2 mR/h) and hence has no risk of exposure.

Command The first component of the incident command system (ICS), responsible for all incident oversight and management. It is the only position in the ICS that must always be staffed.

Command staff The public information officer, safety officer, and liaison officer; they report directly to the incident commander.

Compartment syndrome The clinical findings noted from ischemia and compromised circulation that can occur from vascular injury, causing hypoxia of muscles in an extremity compartment. The cellular edema produces increased pressure in a closed fascial or bony compartment.

Comprehensive emergency management The steps needed to manage an incident, consisting of five components: mitigation, preparedness, response, recovery, and prevention.

Concealment An area or object that hides a person from an assailant's line of sight.

Contact precautions Precautions recommended to reduce the likelihood of transmission of microorganisms by direct or indirect contact.

Contingency care Care that is functionally equivalent to conventional care (e.g., using a different medicine to accomplish the same goal).

Conventional care Care that focuses on doing the best for each individual patient.

Cover A barrier that provides protection from a projectile by stopping or deflecting it.

Crew resource management (CRM) Training procedures designed to optimize performance and outcomes by reducing the effect of human error by using all available resources.

Crisis care Occurs when resource shortfalls cannot be addressed without the risk of poor outcomes for individual patients.

Crisis standards of care (CSC) A substantial change in usual health care operations and the level of care that can be delivered that occurs when a disaster results in *sustained* resource shortages that are severe enough to require changing how health care is delivered across a region.

Decontamination Reduction or removal of hazardous chemical, biologic, or radiologic agents.

Designated incident facilities Assigned locations where specific ICS functions are performed; for example, incident command is located at the incident command post.

Direct threat zone The hot zone in ASHE situations.

Disaster A sudden, calamitous event that seriously disrupts the functioning of a community or society and causes human, material, and economic or environmental losses that exceed the community's or society's ability to cope using its own resources.

Disaster medical assistance teams (DMATs) Teams of specially trained and equipped personnel who provide field care as well as augment existing emergency medical facilities when local resources have been overwhelmed.

Dose rate A measurement of how fast radiation energy is deposited; also known as rate of exposure.

Droplet precautions Precautions recommended to reduce the likelihood of microorganisms transmitted by large droplets expelled by an infected person during talking, sneezing, or coughing or during routine procedures such as suctioning.

Droplet spread Infectious disease transmission through relatively larger infectious aerosols generated from actions such as coughing, breathing, or sneezing.

Emergency medical dispatcher (EMD) A professional telecommunicator who receives emergency assistance calls and is the first step in the EMS resource delivery system.

Endemic An infectious disease that can be regularly found within a community at a given baseline (e.g., chickenpox, herpes).

Epidemic A disease outbreak in which many people in a community or region become infected with the same disease.

Evacuation The timely and rapid movement of people exposed to actual/imminent danger in a disaster to safer locations and places of shelter in order to protect them.

Evacuation corridor An area transitioning between the warm and cold zone, secured from immediate threat allowing for a mitigated risk in transporting victims from the casualty collection points to the triage/treatment area beyond the outer perimeter.

Evacuation warning The alert issued to people in an affected area of a potential threat to life and property.

Finance/administration section Part of the ICS responsible for the accounting and financial aspects of an incident, as well as any legal/policy/regulatory issues that may arise in its aftermath.

Force protection Actions taken by law enforcement to prevent or mitigate hostile actions against personnel, resources, facilities, and critical infrastructures.

Full-thickness (third-degree) burns Burns that involve complete epidermis and dermis.

Gamma ray A ray of high-energy electromagnetic radiation released as a result of radioactive material decay.

Green zone See *cold zone*.

Hazardous material (hazmat) Any substance that poses an unreasonable threat to health, safety, or environment.

High-order explosives (HE) A type of explosive designed to detonate and release its energy very quickly; capable of producing a shock wave, or overpressure phenomenon, that can result in primary blast injury.

Hot zone Also called the red zone, it is the area that poses an immediate danger to life and health (IDLH).

ICS general staff The chiefs of each of the four major sections of the ICS: operations, planning, logistics, and finance/administration.

Immediate evacuation order An order requiring the immediate movement of people out of an affected area due to an imminent threat to life.

Improvised nuclear device (IND) A nuclear weapon constructed from illegally obtained nuclear materials.

Incident action plan (IAP) A continuously updated outline of the overall strategy, tactics, and risk management plans developed by the incident commander or the ICS staff.

Incident command post The location at which incident command functions are performed.

Incident command system (ICS) A system that defines the chain of command and organization of the various resources that respond during a disaster.

Incident commander (IC) The individual responsible for all aspects of a response to an incident.

Indirect threat zone Also called the warm zone in case of ASHE situations, it is an area of relative safety (but not completely secure) where most triage is performed.

Integrated communications A communications system that allows all responders at an incident to communicate with supervisors and subordinates.

LCAN An acronym for **L**ocation, **C**onditions, **A**ctions, and **N**eeds that covers the basic information required for reporting a scene size-up.

Level A PPE The PPE that offers the highest level of respiratory and skin protection. It includes a self-contained breathing apparatus (SCBA) or supplied air respirator (SAR) and a chemical-resistant barrier completely encapsulating the wearer, protecting the skin and mucous membranes.

Level B PPE The PPE that affords the highest respiratory protection, with a lower skin protection level than level A PPE.

Level C PPE The PPE that offers less respiratory protection than level B but similar skin protection.

Level D PPE The PPE that provides minimal respiratory protection and minimal skin protection. It includes standard work clothes and may include a gown, gloves, and surgical mask.

Liaison officer The ICS command staff member who assists or coordinates with multiple agencies; serves as an intermediary between the incident commander and outside agencies.

Logistics section The section responsible for providing all services, equipment, and facilities for an incident.

Low-order explosive (LE) A type of explosive that changes relatively slowly from a solid or liquid to a gaseous state.

Maritime search-and-rescue teams Search-and-rescue teams deployed during hurricanes and in situations involving offshore emergencies.

MARCH A mnemonic that summarizes the clinical treatment priorities in the indirect threat or warm zone—**M**assive hemorrhage control, **A**irway support, **R**espiratory threats, **C**irculation, **H**ypothermia/**H**ead injury.

Mass-casualty incident (MCI) An incident that produces a large number of victims from one mechanism, at one place, and at the same time; also referred to as multiple-casualty incident. It is any incident in which resources are overwhelmed by the number and severity of casualties.

Mass-fatality incident (MFI) A situation in which more fatal accidents occur than can be managed by local resources.

Material safety data sheet (MSDS) A form that provides instructions for the safe handling and storage of a chemical and outlines emergency actions to take if an exposure occurs.

METHANE A mnemonic used for scene size-up—**M**asscasualty incident; **E**xact location; **T**ype of incident; **H**azards present; **A**ccess and egress; **N**umber of casualties and severity; and **E**mergency services required.

Mitigation One of the five components of comprehensive emergency management that happens in the time between disasters, during which plans for response to potential events are developed and tested and actions are taken to prevent or reduce the loss of life through structural and nonstructural measures.

National Incident Management System (NIMS) A standardized structure designed to enable all jurisdictional levels to work collaboratively to manage incident response.

National Urban Search & Rescue (US&R) Response System A framework for organizing federal, state, and local partner advanced technical rescue teams as integrated federal disaster response task forces.

Natural disaster Significant harm to a community following a natural hazard.

Natural hazard An environmental phenomenon that will likely negatively impact societies and the human environment.

Nerve agents Toxic agents that disrupt nerve transmission in the central and peripheral nervous systems by inhibiting acetylcholinesterase, exciting the cholinergic response, and overstimulating the parasympathetic nervous system.

No-notice natural disasters Natural disasters that cannot be predicted, such as earthquakes, volcanic activity, wildfires, avalanches, lightning, and tsunamis.

Nuclear radiation Comprises particles and energy released when atoms break up (fission) or combine (fusion).

Operations section The incident command section responsible for all tactical operations at an incident.

Outbreak An increase in the number of infected people in a limited geographic area.

Outer perimeter The geographic boundary that defines the "safe zone" where no threat should exist at a hazardous incident.

Overpressure phenomenon The sudden increase in atmospheric pressure or shock wave that occurs in proximity to the detonation of a high explosive.

Pandemic A widespread outbreak of an infectious disease that spreads across an entire country or multiple countries.

Person-to-person contact Infectious disease transmission through kissing, sexual intercourse, other body surface contact, or exchange of bodily fluids.

Planning section The ICS section responsible for the collection and evaluation of information related to the incident.

Powered air-purifying respirator (PAPR) A protective respiratory device that draws ambient air through a filter canister and delivers it under positive pressure to a face mask or hood.

Preparedness A step of comprehensive emergency management that involves identifying, in advance of an incident, the specific supplies, equipment, and personnel that would be needed to manage an incident, as well as the specific action plan that would be taken if an incident were to occur.

Prevention A step of comprehensive emergency management that refers to proactively identifying potential hazards and implementing protection measures that could reduce the impact of a disaster.

Primary blast injury Injury that results from high-order explosive detonation and the interaction of the blast overpressure wave with the body or tissue to produce stress and shear waves.

Primary contamination Exposure to a hazardous substance at its point of release.

Psychological first aid (PFA) An evidence-informed approach built on the concept of human resilience that aims to reduce stress symptoms and assist in a healthy recovery following a traumatic event/disaster.

Public information officer (PIO) The ICS command staff officer responsible for interacting with the public and media and distributing information.

Quaternary effects Burns and toxicities from fuel and metals, trauma from structural collapse, and septic syndromes from soil and environmental contamination of wounds following the blast.

Quinary effects Injuries caused by radiation, chemicals, or biologic agents and projectiles such as bone fragments of a suicide bomber.

Radiologic dispersal device (RDD) A conventional explosive device with radiologic contaminants present, or any device that can disperse radioactive material without a nuclear detonation.

Radiologic exposure device (RED) A simple radiologic device designed to expose people to radiation.

Radiologic incendiary device (RID) A radiologic device pairing fire with radioactive contamination.

Recovery One of the five components of comprehensive emergency management that involves the actions necessary to return the community to its preincident functional status.

Red zone See *hot zone*.

Rescue task force A unit of mixed resources, often incorporating law enforcement and prehospital personnel, trained to respond to an active shooter/hostile assailant event.

Resource management Agreements and procedures that enable local, state, and federal agencies to work together under one command during a large-scale incident.

Response One of the five components of comprehensive emergency management that involves activating and deploying the resources to manage an active incident.

Safety officer The ICS command staff officer who is responsible for monitoring, assessing, and ensuring the safety of emergency personnel.

SALT triage Sort, Assess, Lifesaving interventions, Treatment/Transport (SALT), a triage system that is a national guideline for handling MCIs.

Search-and-rescue Effort during a disaster intended to identify and evacuate casualties from the impacted site to a safer location.

Secondary blast injury Injury caused by flying debris and bomb fragments and debris carried by the blast wind resulting in penetrating and blunt trauma.

Secondary contamination Exposure to a hazardous substance after it has been carried away from the point of origin by a victim, a responder, or a piece of equipment.

Secondary devices Explosive devices that may be placed at the scene of an incident, set to explode after the arrival of emergency responders, with the intention of increasing injury, confusion, and panic.

Secondary triage A more detailed assessment performed when the patient arrives at the treatment/transport area.

Self-contained breathing apparatus (SCBA) A personal protective device consisting of a mask and portable supply of air, used in environments that are oxygen-deficient or pose a risk of toxic inhalation.

Shear Change-of-speed force resulting in a cutting or tearing of body parts.

Shear force Energy applied to the body that tends to move an organ or part of the body in one direction while the adjacent part moves in a different direction or remains fixed in place.

Shear wave See *shear force*.

Sheltering in place Selecting a safe space at the current location (work, home, school) and taking refuge there.

Shock wave The boundary between the blast overpressure wave created by a high explosive detonation and normal atmospheric pressure.

Single command A command structure in which a single individual is responsible for all of the strategic objectives of the incident. Typically used when an incident is within a single jurisdiction and is managed by a single discipline.

Situational awareness Involves constant vigilance, in other words paying close and full attention to potential threats and all aspects of the surrounding environment, continuously monitoring the situation for changes, and making good decisions in response to what is observed or sensed.

Source control Controlling the spread of potentially infectious material at the source.

Span of control In an ICS, the number of subordinates who report to one supervisor at any level within the response organization.

Special medical needs shelters Shelters designed to keep displaced noninstitutionalized individuals who need assistance with activities of daily living out of a hospital setting during an emergency.

Spontaneous volunteers Neighbors and ordinary citizens who arrive on site of a disaster ready to help. They may or may not have training and experience related to the disaster.

Staging area A predetermined area where resources, equipment, and personnel can be located safely and at the ready for assignment.

Standard precautions Precautions required when treating all blood and bodily fluid as potentially infectious.

START triage algorithm Simple Triage And Rapid Treatment. A method of evaluating patients and assigning priority for treatment and transport during a mass-casualty incident; involves evaluating the respiratory status, perfusion status, and mental status of the patient.

Supplied air respirator (SAR) A personal protective device consisting of a mask, hose, and compressed air device; used in environments that are oxygen-deficient or pose a risk of toxic inhalation.

Tactical EMS (TEMS) A specialized role for EMS clinicians who support high-risk law enforcement tactical units and train alongside law enforcement officers in drills, communications, and mission planning.

Tertiary blast injury Injury caused by the blast wind throwing the victim's body, resulting in tumbling and collisions with stationary objects.

Toxidrome A collection of clinical signs and symptoms that suggest exposure to a certain class of chemicals or toxins.

Triage French word meaning "to sort"; a process in which a group of patients is sorted according to their priority of need for care.

Triage officer An individual trained to oversee the process of assigning injury severity categories and prioritization of treatment and transport.

Unified command An ICS command structure in which the incident commanders of all the various agencies responding to an event work together to manage the incident.

Unity of command An ICS management concept in which each responder has only one direct supervisor.

Urban search-and-rescue teams Search-and-rescue teams that have advanced training in structural collapse rescue, hazardous materials, and rigging and shoring.

Vapor A solid or liquid in a gaseous state, usually visible as a fine cloud or mist.

Vector-borne transmission Infectious disease transmission when an infectious organism is introduced to a human by an intermediate carrier or reservoir.

Vehicle-borne transmission Infectious disease transmission through items, including biologic materials, that are not necessarily infectious but may transmit infectious pathogens.

Vesicant A chemical agent that causes blistering, such as sulfur mustard and lewisite.

Viral hemorrhagic fever (VHF) A clinical syndrome caused by several different viruses; typified by the clinical presentation of fever, malaise, and hemorrhagic symptoms.

Volatility The likelihood that solids or liquids will vaporize into a gaseous form at room temperature.

Warm zone Also called the yellow zone, it is an area where the concentration of the offending agent is limited and to which victims are brought from the hot zone.

Warned natural disasters Certain natural hazards that can be detected prior to occurring.

Warning A notice that a severe weather event is present in the area.

Watch A notice that conditions exist and are favorable for a severe weather event.

Water rescue teams Rescue teams that have personnel with specialized training and equipment that may include small boat operators, rescue swimmers, and swift water rescue technicians.

Weapon of mass destruction (WMD) A chemical, biologic, radiologic, or explosive agent designed to create significant damage and large numbers of casualties.

White phosphorus An incendiary agent used in the production of munitions.

Wilderness search-and-rescue teams Search-and-rescue teams deployed in cases of uncontrolled wildfires, landslides, avalanches, volcanic eruptions, and lost persons (e.g., hikers lost in the woods).

Yellow zone See *warm zone*.

INDEX

Note: Page numbers followed by *f* and *t* indicate material in figures and tables, respectively.

A

abdominal injuries, 109
active shooter, 34
active shooter/hostile event, 34–38
    basics of zones of care, 35
    clinical treatment priorities, 35–38
    massive hemorrhage, 35–36
    personal protection of EMS during, 34–35
acute radiation syndrome, 94*t*
aerosol precautions, 60
air-purifying respirator (APR), 83
airborne transmission, 58
All Hazards Disaster Response (AHDR)
        course, objectives of, 1
ambulance modification, 64, 65*f*
anthrax, 68–69

B

ballistic vests, 35
barotrauma, 105
biologic agents, 57
bioterrorism, 64–66, 66*t*
    EMS practitioners and, 66–67, 66*f*
bioterrorism agents
    category A, 66
    category B, 66
    category C, 66
blast injuries, types of, 106–107
blast lung injury (BLI), 107–109
blast wave, 106
blast wind, 106
blister agent/vesicant, 85
blunt trauma, 49–50
botulinum toxin, 72

C

casualty collection point, 24
chemical disasters. *See also* radiologic/nuclear
        disasters
    chemical agents, classification of, 85, 86*t*
    decontamination
        ambulatory *vs.* nonambulatory
            patients, 85

        designated decontamination
            areas/corridors, 84
        two-step process, 84–85
    EMS considerations in management, 88–89
        nerve agent, 89–90
        pulmonary agents/lung toxicants, 90–91
        vesicant agents, 91–92
    overview, 85
    personal protective equipment, 83–84, 83*t*
    scene safety
        approaching the hazmat scene, 80
        chemical placards, 80, 80*f*, 83
        hazmat incident identification, 79, 80
        regulatory agency notification, 82
        time of dispatch, 80
    specialized decontamination
        agents, 87–88
    transport considerations in, 92
    type of exposure
        ingestion, 87
        injection, 87
        oral and inhalation, 87
    volatility of chemical agent, 87
    zones of operation, 82, 83*f*
chemical placards, 80, 80*f*
clinical treatment priorities, MCI and, 35–38
    cold zone, 38
    direct threat/hot zone, 35
    indirect threat/warm zone, 36–38
        airway management, 37
        circulation, 38
        head injury, 38
        hypothermia, 38
        massive hemorrhage, 36–37
        respirations, 37–38
cold zone, 20
    clinical treatment priorities, 38
command staff, 10–11
command, defined, 9
compartment syndrome, 110–111
comprehensive emergency management,
        4–5, 4*f*
    mitigation, 4
    preparedness, 4
    prevention, 4
    recovery, 5

    response, 5
concealment, 35
contact precautions, 59
contingency care, 15
control zones, 19–20, 19*f*
    cold zone, 20
    dynamic nature of, 20
    hot zone, 19
    warm zone, 19–20
conventional care, 15
cover, 35
crew resource management (CRM), 26
crisis care, 15
crisis standards of care (CSC), 15
crush injuries/crush syndrome, 50

D

decontamination, 64
    hazmat disasters
        ambulatory *vs.* nonambulatory
            patients, 85
        designated decontamination
            areas/corridors, 84
        two-step process, 84–85
designated incident facilities, 9
direct threat zone, 19
    clinical treatment priorities, 35
disaster, 2*f*
    and emergency medical response.
        See emergency medical response
    bioterrorism and, 64–66, 66*t*
    comprehensive emergency management,
        4–5, 4*f*
        mitigation, 4
        preparedness, 4
        prevention, 4
        recovery, 5
        response, 5
    description of, 1–2
    specialty response teams, 12–15
        disaster medical assistance teams, 14
        spontaneous volunteers, 12
        types of, 12–13
    tactical EMS, 13–14
    types of, 2–3

disaster (*Continued*)
  hazmat disasters, 3
  infectious diseases and biologic
    disasters, 3
  mass-casualty incidents, 2, 3*f*
  natural disaster, 3, 3*f*
  weapon of mass destruction disasters, 3
disaster medical assistance teams (DMATs),
  14, 15*f*
doffing of PPE, 62, 64, 62*f*–63*f*
donning of PPE, 62, 64, 62*f*–63*f*
dose rate meters, 96
droplet precautions, 59
droplet spread, 58

E

Ebola virus, 71–72
emergency medical dispatchers (EMDs), 33
emergency medical response, 17–28
  control zones, 19–20, 19*f*
    cold zone, 20
    dynamic nature of, 20
    hot zone, 19
    warm zone, 19–20
  goals, 17
  initial response, 17–18, 18*f*
  practitioners, physical impact of, 27
  psychological response, 26–27
    factors impacting, 26–27
    interventions, 27
    signs of psychological trauma, 27
  retriage, 25
  safety principles, 25–26
    crew resource management, 26
    situational awareness, 25–26
  transport, 25
    means of transport, 25
    patient/transport destination, 25
  triage and treatment, 20–25
    casualty collection points, 24
    categories, 23–24, 23*f*
    dynamic process, 25
    methodologies, 20–22, 21*f*, 22*f*
    procedures performed during, 24
EMS management, 68–72
  anthrax, 68–69
  botulinum toxin, 72
  chemical disasters, 88
    nerve agent, 89–90
    pulmonary agents/lung toxicants,
      90–91
    vesicant agents, 91–92
  Ebola virus, 71–72
  plague, 69
  small pox, 69–71, 70*f*
EMS response, infectious diseases and
  biologic disasters, 66–68
  biologic emergencies, 67

concentrated biohazard agent *vs.* infected
  patient, 67
  steps to prevent infection, 67–68
endemic, 57, 57*f*
Environmental Protection Agency (EPA), 82
epidemic, 57, 57*f*
evacuation, 43
evacuation corridor, 35
evacuation warning, 43
explosions, 31
  causes of, 103
  closed- *vs.* open-space, 103
  law enforcement interface, 104
  situational awareness, 104
  special populations, 105
  terminology, 106
  transport considerations, 105
  triage considerations, 104–105
explosives, categories of, 105–106

F

finance/administration section, 11
force protection, 34

G

gamma rays, 93
general staff, ICS, 11
green zone, 20

H

hazardous material (hazmat), 79
  classes of, 81*t*–82*t*
hazmat disasters, 3
head injuries, 38, 109–110
hemorrhage, 35–36
high-order explosives (HE), 105
hot zone, 19
hydroxocobalamin, 89
hypothermia, 38

I

immediate evacuation order, 44
improvised nuclear device (IND), 95
incendiary agents, 111
  magnesium, 111
  thermite, 111
  white phosphorus, 111
incident action plan (IAP), 8
incident command post, 10
incident commander, 9, 10*f*
incident management system (IMS), 7–16
  advantages of, 7
  characteristics, 8
    all-hazards system, 8
    common terminology, 8
    designated incident facilities, 9

    incident action plan, 8
    integrated communications, 8
    resource management, 8
    span of control, 8
    unity of command, 8
  managing and preserving resources, 15
  organization of, 9–12, 9*f*
    command staff, 10–11
    general staff, 11–12
    incident command post, 10
    single *vs.* unified command, 9–12
  overview, 7
indirect threat zone, 20
  clinical treatment priorities, 36–38
infectious diseases and biologic disasters,
  3, 57–76
  ambulance modification, 64, 65*f*
  bioterrorism, 64–66, 66*t*
    EMS practitioners and, 66–67, 66*f*
  case study, 73–76
  considerations, 57–64
  controlling infectious disease
    transmission, 59–60, 59*f*
  disease outbreak terminology, 57
  EMS management, 68–72
    anthrax, 68–69
    botulinum toxin, 72
    Ebola virus, 71–72
    plague, 69
    small pox, 69–71, 70*f*
  EMS practitioners, bioterrorism and,
    66–67
  EMS response, 65–68
    biologic emergencies, 67
    concentrated biohazard agent *vs.*
      infected patient, 67
    steps to prevent infection, 67–68
  models of infectious disease transmission,
    58–59, 58*f*
  pandemic preparedness and response, 73
  personal protective equipment, 60–64,
    61*f*–63*f*
    donning and doffing, 62, 64, 62*f*–63*f*
    fit testing, 60
    types of, 60–62, 61*f*
integrated communications, 8

L

LCAN Report, 18
lethal triad, 38*f*
liaison officer, 11
logistics section, 11
low-order explosives (HE), 105

M

magnesium, 111
MARCH mnemonic, 36
maritime search-and-rescue teams, 13, 14*f*

mass-casualty incident (MCI), 2, 3f, 29–38
  active shooter/hostile event, 34–38
    basics of zones of care, 35
    clinical treatment priorities, 35–38
    personal protection of EMS during, 34–35
  description of, 29
  EMS response priorities, 29–30
  fatality management, 30
    biologic disasters, clinical issues, 30
  patients with special needs, 30–31
  rural settings, EMS challenges in, 31
  transportation, 33, 34f
  urban settings, EMS challenges in, 31–33
mass-fatality incident (MFI), 39
material safety data sheets (MSDS), 82
mechanisms of injury
  abdominal injuries, 109
  blast injuries, types of, 106–107
  blast Lung Injury (BLI), 107–109
  compartment syndrome, 110–111
  head injuries, 109–110
  multisystem trauma, 110
  tympanic membrane rupture, 109
METHANE, 18
multisystem trauma, 110

N

National Incident Management System (NIMS), 7
National Urban Search & Rescue (US&R) Response System, 14
natural disaster, 3, 3f, 41
  common injuries, 49–50
    blunt trauma, 49–50
    crush injuries/crush syndrome, 50
    exacerbation of medical conditions, 50
    orthopedic injuries, 50
  evacuation, 43–45
    phases of, 43–44, 45f
    psychological and social impact, 43
    sheltering in place and, 44–45
  local populations, 48–49, 49f
  no-notice, 42
  patient tracking, 51
  potential hazards for EMS, 48–49
  preparedness, 50–54
    emergency supply list, 52–53
    first aid kit, 54
    food kit, 53
    personal, 51
  public education, 51
  triage and transport, 50
  vulnerable patients/special needs population, 45–48
    caregivers and chaperons, 46
    communication, 46
    destination determination, 47–48

    identifying, 47
    maintaining independence, 45–46
    medical care, 46
    transportation, 46
    warned, 41–42
  natural hazard, 41
nerve agents, 89–90
no-notice natural disasters, 42
nuclear radiation, 92

O

Occupational Safety and Health Administration (OSHA), 82, 87
operations section, 11
orthopedic injuries, 50
outbreak, 57
outer perimeter, 35
overpressure phenomenon, 105

P

pandemic, 57, 57f
person-to-person contact, 58
personal protective equipment (PPE), 60–64, 61f–63f
  chemical disasters, 83–84, 83t
  donning and doffing, 62, 64, 62f–63f
  fit testing, 60
  level A, 60, 62, 61f
  level B, 62, 61f
  level C, 61f, 62
  level D, 61f, 62
  radiologic/nuclear disasters, 83–84, 83t
  types of, 60–62, 61f
plague, 69
planning section, 11
powered air-purifying respirator (PAPR), 71
primary blast injuries, 106
primary contamination, 87
psychological first aid (PFA), 27
psychological response, emergency medical response and, 26–27
  factors impacting, 26–27
  interventions, 27
  signs of psychological trauma, 27
public information officer (PIO), 11

Q

quaternary effects, 107
quinary effects, 107

R

radiation exposure
  diagnosing, 95
  dose rate meters, 96
  prevention of untoward effects, 95–96

  understandings of, 95
radiologic dispersal device (RDD), 95
radiologic exposure device (RED), 95
radiologic incendiary device (RID), 95
radiologic weapons, types of, 95
  improvised nuclear device, 95
  radiologic dispersal device, 95
  radiologic exposure device, 95
  radiologic incendiary device, 95
radiologic/nuclear disasters. *See also* chemical disasters
  decontamination
    ambulatory *vs.*nonambulatory patients, 84
    designated decontamination areas/corridors, 84
    two-step process, 84–85
  disaster scenarios, 93, 95
  overview, 92
  personal protective equipment, 83–84, 83t
  principles of management and decontamination, 96
  radiation exposure
    diagnosing, 95
    dose rate meters, 96
    prevention of untoward effects, 95–96
    understandings of, 95
  radiologic weapons, types of, 95
    improvised nuclear device, 95
    radiologic dispersal device, 95
    radiologic exposure device, 95
    radiologic incendiary device, 95
  scene safety
    approaching the hazmat scene, 80
    chemical placards, 80, 80f, 83
    hazmat incident identification, 79, 80
    regulatory agency notification, 82
    time of dispatch, 80
  transport considerations, 96
  types of ionizing radiation
    gamma rays, 94
    nuclear radiation, 92–93
  zones of operation, 82, 83f
red zone, 19
rescue task force, 35
resource management, 9

S

safety officer, 11
SALT triage, 21–22, 21f
search-and-rescue, 12
secondary blast injuries, 107
secondary contamination, 87
secondary devices, 104
self-contained breathing apparatus (SCBA), 60
shear forces, 49
shear waves, 106
sheltering in place, 44–45

shock wave, 106
Simple Triage and Rapid Treatment (START),
    20, 21*f*
single command, 8, 9–10
situational awareness, 25
small pox, 69–71, 70*f*
source control, 59
span of control, 8
special medical needs shelters, 48
spontaneous volunteers, 12
staging area, 9
standard precautions, 59
supplied air respirator (SAR), 60*t*

T

tactical EMS (TEMS), 13–14
tertiary blast injuries, 107
thermite, 111
toxidrome, 85, 86*t*
transport considerations
    chemical disasters, 92
    emergency medical response, 25
    emergency medical response and, 25
        means of transport, 25
        patient/transport destination, 25

explosions, 105
    mass-casualty incident, 33, 34*f*
    natural disaster, 46
    radiologic/nuclear disasters, 96
triage, 20
    emergency medical response and, 20–25
        casualty collection points, 24
        categories, 23–24, 23*f*
        dynamic process, 25
        methodologies, 20–22, 21*f*, 22*f*
        procedures performed during, 24
    explosions, 104–105
triage officer, 20
tympanic membrane rupture, 109

U

unified command, 8
unity of command, 8
urban search-and-rescue teams, 12–13

V

vapor, 84
vector-borne transmission, 58
vehicle-borne transmission, 59

viral hemorrhagic fever, 71
volatility, 87
vulnerable patients/special needs
        population, natural disaster
        and, 45–48
    caregivers and chaperons, 46
    communication, 46
    destination determination, 47–48
    identifying, 47
    maintaining independence, 45–46
    medical care, 46
    transportation, 46

W

warm zone, 19–20
warned natural disasters, 41–42
warning, 41–42, 43*f*
watch, 42, 43*f*
water rescue teams, 13, 14*f*
weapon of mass destruction (WMD), 3, 67
white phosphorus, 111
wilderness search-and-rescue teams, 13, 13*f*

Y

yellow zone, 19–20

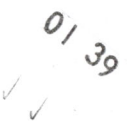